Psychological Treatment
of
Chronic
Illness

Psychological Treatment
of
Chronic
Illness

The Biopsychosocial Therapy Approach

Len Sperry, MD, PhD

American Psychological Association • Washington, DC

Published by
American Psychological Association
750 First Street, NE
Washington, DC 20002
www.apa.org

To order
APA Order Department
P.O. Box 92984
Washington, DC 20090-2984
Tel: (800) 374-2721; Direct: (202) 336-5510
Fax: (202) 336-5502; TDD/TTY: (202) 336-6123
Online: www.apa.org/books/
E-mail: order@apa.org

In the U.K., Europe, Africa, and the Middle East, copies may be ordered from
American Psychological Association
3 Henrietta Street
Covent Garden, London
WC2E 8LU England

Typeset in Palatino by Stephen McDougal, Mechanicsville, MD

Printer: Data Reproductions, Auburn Hills, MI
Cover Designer: Naylor Design, Washington, DC
Technical/Production Editor: Devon Bourexis

The opinions and statements published are the responsibility of the authors, and such opinions and statements do not necessarily represent the policies of the American Psychological Association.

Library of Congress Cataloging-in-Publication Data

Sperry, Len.
   Psychological treatment of chronic illness : the biopsychosocial therapy approach / Len Sperry.—1st ed.
      p. cm.
   Includes bibliographical references and index.
   ISBN 1-59147-354-3
   1. Chronic diseases—Psychological aspects. 2. Chronic diseases—Social aspects.
3. Psychotherapy. 4. Clinical health psychology. I. Title.

   RC108.S68 2005
   616'.001'9—dc22   2005020258

British Library Cataloguing-in-Publication Data
A CIP record is available from the British Library.

Printed in the United States of America
First Edition

CONTENTS

FOREWORD

In these early years of the 21st century, we are witnessing dramatic improvements in health care science and technology. However, the overall picture for health care is not good. Health care costs continue to escalate faster than those of other segments of the economy, and the number of uninsured has now passed 45 million Americans. The Institute of Medicine (2002) recently concluded that "the health care delivery system is incapable of meeting the present, let alone the future needs of the American public" (p. 1).

These problems are clearly so serious that they should compel a complete reexamination of the U.S. health care system. One core assumption that requires rethinking is the idea of the separation of mind from body, the notion pervading our concepts of health and illness that there are some illnesses that are physical and others that are mental, a notion that informs the current practice in health care reimbursement of subcapitating mental health benefits. As we all know, mind and body are not separate, but rather they are inseparable. By assuming that mind and body are separate, and further, assuming that the only role that the mind plays in health and illness is in mental health and illness, we have maintained a health care system that is unable to deal with the many varied roles that mind and behavior play in so-called physical illness. Further, this system does not even deal with mental health and illness, per se, effectively.

Descartes's 17th-century metaphysical philosophy, which separates mind from body, has had an enormously negative impact on our health care system. Because of it, our health care system does not systematically attend to the many psychological risk factors for both morbidity and mortality, and it

This foreword is adapted from "Health Care for the Whole Person," by R. F. Levant, 2005, *APA Monitor on Psychology, 36*, p. 5. Copyright 2005 by the American Psychological Association.

virtually ignores the psychosocial pathways that lead to unnecessary use of medical and surgical services. Further, our health care system does not fully use appropriate tools to tackle the current chronic disease epidemic, such as the numerous disease management programs aimed at treatment adherence and lifestyle improvement developed and validated by psychologists. Nor does it use fully the many well-documented psychological interventions for acute illness and management of stressful medical procedures. In addition, the psychological impact of having a medical illness is not well addressed by the health care system, nor is the fact that many people who have a physical illness also have a comorbid psychological illness, nor is prescription drug abuse. Finally, the lion's share of mental health problems are treated, ineffectively, by primary care providers.

Mind–body dualism, is, in a word, bankrupt. We need to transform our biomedical health care system to one based on the biopsychosocial model, which will emphasize collaboration between medical and behavioral health care providers and the integration of psychology into the very heart of health care. To reform the U.S. health care system along these lines, we must appeal directly to the public and to decision makers, not alone, but in collaboration with other like-minded physician, provider, consumer, and policy groups. We need to articulate the public's dissatisfaction with the biomedical health care system that results from care providers not having time to listen to all of their concerns or offering ineffective care. We need to put forth a vision of integrated care, a care system that offers health care for the whole person.

Psychologists and other psychotherapists will have an enormous role to play in this transformed health care system, particularly in the area of chronic disease. Chronic disease is enormous, affecting 50% of the population now and threatening to get larger as the baby-boom generation enters old age. Yet few mental health practitioners have been trained to work with patients who have chronic illnesses. Hence, this volume, *Psychological Treatment of Chronic Illness: The Biopsychosocial Therapy Approach*, could not be more timely.

I have occasion to speak before groups of psychologists at state psychological associations and other types of meetings and have found that many established practitioners are still reeling from the devastating effects of managed care, and early career psychologists are struggling to get on panels. I have suggested that some consider the idea of establishing a practice in the area of chronic illness. I point out that they would need some additional education, through continuing education or self-study, and perhaps supervised experience if they have never trained or worked in a medical setting. But I also note that I do not think that most would need to do a formal postdoctoral year in clinical health psychology or medical family therapy if they were to focus on one or two highly prevalent chronic illnesses, such as diabetes or hypertension. I suggest that they could locate their practice in a medical office building, which would greatly facilitate marketing their services to physicians. Practitioners, I note, could use the new health and behavior procedure codes that have been approved by the Center for Medicaid and Medicare Services, which allows practitioners to bill Medicare and a growing number of commercial carriers for psychological assessment and psychotherapy with patients under an _ICD–9 medical diagnosis._ Now when I give these talks, I will also strongly urge that they consult Len Sperry's enormously helpful new book!

Ronald F. Levant
Health Care for the Whole Person
University of Akron

PREFACE

According to the National Center for Chronic Disease Prevention and Health Promotion (2000), statistics on chronic diseases are daunting: Ninety million Americans have one or more of these diseases, and 70% of all deaths are attributed to them. It is difficult to fathom that 75% of adults age 65 and older have diabetes and that 1,700 new cases of diabetes are diagnosed every day. Compared with prevalence rates of mental illness, the prevalence of chronic disease is at least 3 times higher. Statistics on children are equally daunting: Thirty percent of all children have these diseases (Meyer & Lewis, 1994).

With the average life span now extending into the 80s, the reality is that most people will experience chronic illness in themselves or in the lives of those close to them. Rather sobering is the fact that health care professionals, including psychotherapists, will experience chronic illness and disability for which they will receive care from others. It seems difficult to imagine the practice of psychotherapy in which many, if not most, patients who present with obvious psychological issues will also be experiencing a chronic medical illness. That means that whether clinically oriented psychologists and other psychotherapists focus their practice primarily on treating chronic illness or whether they focus on providing conventional psychotherapeutic services, they will all be involved with chronic illness.

Today, unfortunately, health care professionals seem to have little to offer those who present with chronic diseases, as witnessed by the increasing patient dissatisfaction with conventional medicine. Why is this? In large part, it is because the training of health care professionals has primarily emphasized the treatment of acute disease wherein such diseases are viewed as an objective biomedical reality with a single cause and single treatment. However, chronic illness is the subjective experience of chronic disease, and such diseases tend to have multiple causes and treatments. This means that the experience of chronic illness is quite variable, depending on several biopsychosocial factors, including biomedical, personality, coping, and cultural factors.

It is regrettable that the health care system focuses primarily on the biomedical dimension of chronic illness and the psychosocial and cultural dimension are ignored or inadequately addressed. The result is needless suffering and disability. It is likely that the prevalence rates of chronic illness will skyrocket as the population ages. Despite recent recommendations of national commissions and blue-ribbon panels that health professionals be trained in and expected to provide comprehensive biopsychosocial treatment, there has been little change in the training programs or expectations for comprehensive treatment. In short, a major health care crisis looms at a time when organized health care seems unprepared to meet it.

Fortunately, because of their psychosocial training, psychologists and other psychotherapists are well positioned to respond to this major health care challenge. However, to provide effective and appropriate treatment to such patients will require that psychotherapists augment their psychosocial perspective and conventional psychotherapeutic strategies with a biopsychosocial perspective and biopsychosocially oriented treatment strategies. This book emphasizes such a biopsychosocial perspective and describes a biopsychosocially oriented treatment approach, referred to as *Biopsychosocial Therapy*.

Psychological Treatment of Chronic Illness is unique in its focus on the experience of chronic illness from both the patient's and the provider's perspective. It emphasizes the need for, and clinical value of, a comprehensive biopsychosocial assessment, case conceptualization, and treatment plan. It also stresses the value of tailoring the treatment process and sequencing treatment interventions to personality dynamics, family and cultural dynamics, and health dynamics, including illness representation or explanatory model and course and progression of the illness. Additionally, because countertransference is considerably more common in people who are chronically ill than it is in traditional psychotherapy patients, countertransference and other therapeutic relationship issues are addressed as well. Several extended case studies are provided to clarify and illustrate significant points and issues. The extensive use of session transcriptions provides readers with a feel for working with those who are chronically ill in a treatment setting.

Psychological Treatment of Chronic Illness is divided into two parts. Part I introduces and provides a detailed overview of the biopsychosocial perspective on chronic illness. It consists of four chapters. Chapter 1 sketches a panoramic overview of chronic illness and treatment considerations germane to psychotherapists. Then, the need for and clinical value of the biopsychosocial model of chronic illness is discussed in chapter 2 and is contrasted with the biomedical and psychosocial models of illness. Chapter 3 addresses the biopsychosocial aspects of common chronic illnesses. It provides a focused description of both the disease process and the illness experience for 10 common chronic conditions. Finally, chapter 4 discusses the influence of personality dynamics on chronic illness. Six personality types are described in terms of their characteristic personality and health-related dynamics and illness representations and how they typically interact with clinicians and respond to the treatment process. Part II describes and illustrates the Biopsychosocial Therapy approach to chronic illness. It consists of five chapters. Chapter 5 provides a detailed description of the Biopsychosocial Therapy approach, including its history, basic premises, and common clinical indications. It describes its four phases and its process goals and outcome goals in the treatment of chronic illnesses. A signature feature of this approach is a comprehensive biopsychosocial assessment, and chapter 6 describes the assessment process and the way in which cases are conceptualized and treatment is planned, sequenced, and implemented. Chapters 7 through 9 illustrate this assessment and treatment process with actual cases and extensive session transcriptions. Chapter 7 describes an extended first session demonstrating the use of several therapeutic strategies, including a comprehensive assessment and treatment intervention. Chapter 8 highlights the use of the Biopsychosocial Therapy approach with difficult, complex, and so-called treatment-resistant patients who are chronically ill, using intensive psychotherapy strategies. Finally, chapter 9 describes and illustrates the use of health-focused counseling strategies in a patient who is chronically ill and who, although she has not responded to previous biomedical treatments, is quite receptive and responsive to a biopsychosocial approach.

This book addresses the needs of psychologists, psychiatric nurses, social workers, and counselors who collaborate to treat patients who experience chronic illness. Their collaboration as a part of the medical team brings comprehensive care that improves treatment adherence, promotes positive lifestyle changes, and alleviates the stress of medical procedures. In many ways, their collaboration is instrumental to the success of the biopsychosocial model. In addition to this professional audience, the book is written to address the needs of students and trainees in graduate and postgraduate training programs in psychology, counseling, nursing, and health education programs. It is hoped that their work with the biopsychosocial model will bring continued refinements and a higher quality of life to the many people who struggle with chronic illnesses.

ACKNOWLEDGMENTS

The development and completion of this book occurred over the past 3 years, beginning with the video *Chronic Illness* in the American Psychological Association's (APA's) Behavioral Health series. I am particularly grateful to Jon Carlson, host of that series, for the invitation to make the video and to Susan Reynolds, acquisitions editor at APA Books, who encouraged me to develop a book based on that video. My appreciation extends to several colleagues who have been exceedingly generous with their encouragement and friendship: Harry Prosen, MD; Jon Gudeman, MD; Carl Chan, MD; Richard Cox, MD, PhD; and Richard Sauber, PhD. APA Books has, as in the past, been an important collaborator in this venture. My heartfelt appreciation is extended to Julia Frank-McNeil, Susan Reynolds, and Devon Bourexis.

I

A BIOPSYCHOSOCIAL
PERSPECTIVE ON
CHRONIC ILLNESS

1

TREATING CHRONIC ILLNESS:
AN OVERVIEW

Increasingly, patients with chronic diseases are being referred to psychologists and psychotherapists for treatment. Because of the nature of chronic illness, individuals with these disease entities present physicians and other health care providers with incredibly difficult treatment challenges. This is largely because unlike acute illnesses, wherein psychosocial factors have only limited bearing, psychosocial factors are prominent and dominant in chronic illnesses. It is not surprising that clinically oriented psychologists and other psychotherapists have much to offer individuals experiencing chronic illness. This chapter provides a panoramic overview of chronic illness and treatment considerations germane to psychotherapists. The chapter has four main sections. The first provides basic information about chronic disease such as prevalence, types, costs, and basic definitions. The second section describes the experience of chronic illness from the patient's perspective in terms of a phase model. The third section discusses theoretical and therapeutic issues unique to chronic illness. These include wellness and health; cure and healing; pain, suffering, and stigma; and spirituality and religious issues. The fourth section provides an overview of the treatment process and approaches. It briefly describes various forms of health counseling and the dominant treat-

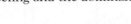

ment approach, with chronic disease, that is, cognitive–behavioral therapy (CBT). It reviews some research on the effectiveness of various approaches to chronic illness and provides a brief glimpse of *Biopsychosocial Therapy*. Finally, it provides a brief overview of subsequent chapters.

CHRONIC DISEASE—A PRIMER

The type of diseases contributing most heavily to death, illness, and disability among Americans changed dramatically during the last century. Today, chronic diseases such as cardiovascular disease (primarily heart disease and stroke), cancer, and diabetes are among the most prevalent, costly, and preventable of all health problems. The prolonged course of illness and disability from chronic diseases such as diabetes and arthritis results in extended pain and suffering and decreased quality of life for millions of Americans.

Chronic, disabling conditions cause major limitations in activity for more than 1 of every 10, or 25 million, Americans. The Centers for Disease Control and Prevention reports that nearly three quarters of adults age 65 years and older have one or more chronic illnesses, and nearly half report two or more (National Center for Chronic Disease Prevention and Health Promotion, 2000). With an aging population, chronic diseases will increase proportionately. Moreover, children and young people who have a chronic disease, such as juvenile-onset diabetes, can expect to live longer and, therefore, will have a need to manage their health condition or conditions over a longer life span than in the past. With an increasing life span, older individuals will require more health services longer for chronic health conditions. Every year, chronic diseases claim the lives of more than 1.7 million Americans. These diseases are responsible for 7 of every 10 deaths in the United States (National Center for Chronic Disease Prevention and Health Promotion, 2000).

What accounts for this increase in chronic diseases? Many answers have been suggested, including the standard American diet—which is characterized by a high intake of simple carbohydrates, such as sugar, and other unhealthy food choices—environmental factors such as exposure to heavy metals like mercury, cadmium, and aluminum, and oxidative stress (Lane, 2003), as well as improvements in medical care itself: Better emergency treatments allow many individuals to survive the initial critical stages of acute illnesses or trauma, such as an accident or heart attack. Individuals live with the effects of these acute illnesses and trauma and thus face chronic illness from which they will never recover. In short, improved acute medical care, together with demographic trends indicating an increase in the elderly population, contributes to an increase in chronic illness (Friedman & DiMatteo, 1989; Goodheart & Lansing, 1996).

Costs of Chronic Disease

The United States cannot effectively address escalating health care costs without addressing the problem of chronic diseases, because more than 90 million Americans—approximately one third of all men, women, and children—live with chronic diseases. As previously noted, chronic diseases account for 70% of deaths in the United States and account for one third of the years of potential life lost before age 65 (Robert Wood Johnson Foundation, 1994).

The cost of health care for individuals with chronic illnesses does not typically take into account the personal, occupational, and financial costs related to self-management or disabilities. Nor does it account for the social and psychological burdens placed on the individual, the family, and society as a whole by the 90 million Americans with one or more chronic diseases (McGinnis, Williams-Russo, & Knickman, 2002). The medical care costs for individuals with chronic diseases total more than $400 billion annually, which is more than 60% of total medical care expenditures (National Center for Chronic Disease Prevention and Health Promotion, 2000).

Prevalence in Women and Racial Minorities

According to the National Center for Chronic Disease Prevention and Health Promotion (2000), chronic disease disproportionately affects women and racial minority populations. Women comprise more than half of the people who die each year of cardiovascular disease. Deaths due to breast cancer are decreasing among Caucasian women but not among African American women. The death rate from cervical cancer is more than twice as high for African American women as it is for Caucasian women. The 5-year survival rate for men with colon cancer is 51% for African Americans and 63% for Caucasians. The prevalence of diabetes is about 1.7 times more among non-Hispanic African Americans, 1.9 times more among Hispanics, and 2.8 times more among American Indian and Alaska Natives than among non-Hispanic White Americans of similar age. The death rate from prostate cancer is more than twice as high for African American men as it is for Caucasian men. African Americans are more likely than Caucasians to get oral or pharyngeal cancer, half as likely to have those diseases diagnosed early, and twice as likely to die of these diseases.

Definition of Terms

Although many use the terms *disease and illness* interchangeably, they actually have quite different meanings. Whereas *disease* represents an objective process, *illness* is a subjective process. The National Center for Chronic

Disease Prevention and Health Promotion (2000) defines *chronic diseases* as those illnesses that are preventable and that pose a significant burden in mortality, morbidity, and cost. It is important to distinguish *disease* from *illness* and *chronic disease* from *chronic illness*. Defining *chronic disease* and *chronic illness* is complex. Lubkin and Larsen (2002) reviewed eight different definitions proposed by national commissions and researchers since 1957. In short, there is no consensus definition. Accordingly, I define the following terms, which are used throughout this book:

Disease: An objective and definable process characterized by pathophysiology and pathology.

Illness: The subjective experience of a disease state.

Acute disease: A disease entity with a single cause, a specific onset, and identifiable symptoms that are often treatable with a single biological intervention—that is, drugs or surgery—and is usually curable.

Chronic disease: A disease entity that usually does not have a single cause, a specific onset, or a stable set of symptoms. Such a disease state is largely an objective entity. Although a cure may be possible for mild levels, it is unlikely for moderate and advanced levels of disease process. The disease course tends to be marked by periods of exacerbation and remission as well as progressive degeneration. Biopsychosocial interventions are commonly used to achieve treatment goals of coping, management, or palliation.

Chronic illness: The subjective experience of a chronic disease.

Classification of Chronic Disease

Because of considerable variability among presentations of the same chronic disease—and even more among chronic illness presentations—there is no consensus about the classification of such a disease state. However, four major types of chronic illnesses can be noted. The first are the life-threatening diseases, such as fast-growing cancers and serious cardiovascular conditions like stroke and heart attacks. Health-focused counseling and psychotherapy with these tend to be emergent and brief. A second type of chronic disease includes the manageable ones, such as Type 2 diabetes, hypertension, osteoarthritis, and chronic sinusitis. Although they may become serious, they are seldom life threatening. Health-focused counseling and psychotherapy of individuals with this second type of chronic disease tends to be a bit longer than, and not quite as emergent as, it is with the first type. The third type includes progressively disabling diseases such as Parkinson's disease, systemic lupus erythematosus, rheumatoid arthritis, and multiple sclerosis. Health-focused counseling and psychotherapy with these can often be similar to ongoing psychotherapy. A fourth type involves those that are not life threatening but that have waxing and waning courses that are sometimes, but not always, debilitating. Examples of this type are chronic fatigue syndrome and fibromyalgia. Health-focused counseling and psychotherapy with these may be longer and emphasize efforts to prevent remissions and symptom amelioration.

THE EXPERIENCE OF CHRONIC ILLNESS

[handwritten: acute]

The experience of having an acute disease, such as the common cold, is easy to describe because, for most people, it has the same symptom presentation and follows a short, predictable course. It begins with nasal congestion and a sore throat, which within a day leads to a feeling of fullness with copious nasal discharge that irritates the nose. After 3 days, the major signs diminish, but the "stuffed-up" feeling may continue for up to a week. During that time, the individual may have a bit less energy. Essentially, symptom, course, and recovery are reasonably consistent and predictable for most people. However, a key characteristic of a chronic illness is its variability in terms of symptom and course, and there may or may not be a recovery phase, depending on the disease and the individual. Although the symptoms of chronic illness are not experienced constantly by everyone, approximately 50% experience their chronic illness constantly (Fennell, 2003). Needless to say, the experience of a chronic illness is much more variable than that of an acute illness. This variability is confusing for clinicians and can complicate both the therapeutic relationship and the treatment process. Despite this variability, researchers have been able to articulate the experience of adjustment to a chronic disease from the patient's perspective in terms of a phase model.

[handwritten: Fennell "phases" 4 phase model]

A Phase Model of Chronic Illness

Fennell (2001, 2003) has described a phase model of chronic illness. She uses the term *phase* rather than *stage* because *stage* implies a forward-moving progression whereas *phase* implies that both progression and regression are possible. These four phases, as listed in the following sections, are based on her clinical research with several hundred patients with a variety of chronic diseases.

Phase 1: Crisis

The onset of illness triggers a crisis for which individuals seek relief through medical diagnosis and treatment, spiritual help, or substance abuse. Family, coworkers, and caregivers may respond with disbelief, revulsion, and rejection. In this phase, the basic task is to deal with the immediate symptoms, pain, or traumas associated with this new experience of illness.

Phase 2: Stabilization

A plateau of symptoms is reached, and individuals become more familiar with their illness. They attempt to carry on their pre-illness activity level, which overtaxes them and contributes to relapses and ensuing feelings of upset and failure. The basic task of this phase is to stabilize and restructure life patterns and perceptions.

Phase 3: Resolution

Amid plateaus of symptoms and relapses, individuals understand their illness pattern and others' response to it. There is initial acceptance that one's pre-illness sense of self will not return. In this phase, the basic task is to develop a new self and to seek a personally meaningful philosophy of life and a spirituality consistent with it.

Phase 4: Integration

Despite plateaus and relapses, individuals are able to integrate parts of their old self before the illness to their new self. In this phase, the basic task is to find appropriate employment if able to work, to reintegrate or form supportive networks of friends and family, and to integrate one's illness within a spiritual or philosophical framework. It also means achieving the highest level of wellness possible despite compromised or failing health. Accordingly, *integration* means coming "to experience a complete life in which illness is only one aspect" (Fennell, 2003, p. 9).

Not every individual with a chronic illness manages to journey through all four stages. As Fennell (2003) pointed out, many individuals who are chronically ill get caught in a recurring loop of cycling between Phase 1 and Phase 2, wherein each crisis produces new wounding and destabilization of the individual's biopsychosocial system. Such crises tend to be followed by a brief period of stabilization, and without intervention, a new crisis invariably destabilizes the system again. With appropriate health-focused counseling, individuals who are chronically ill can be assisted in breaking this recurring cycle and move to Phases 3 and 4.

Some people, particularly those on the margins of society with almost no sources of support, never escape Phase 1. They are buffeted from crisis to crisis, some relieved only by alcohol and drugs. As Fennell (2001) stated, "These individuals often lose everything they have . . . simply because they are sick and have not received the care and help they need" (pp. 40–41).

Thus, appropriate and competent health-focused counseling can help individuals with a chronic illness find a new meaning in life. Besides providing support, it provides patients the needed encouragement and coping skills to live that life with a measure of dignity and a sense of wellness.

Case Example

Jennifer is a 41-year-old married attorney without children. She works in the public defender's office, and her husband is a senior partner in a large accounting firm.

Phase 1

Over several weeks, she notices that she has become increasingly fatigued and unable to concentrate. Nevertheless, she pushes herself with her regular family and work responsibilities despite not feeling well. At a certain point, she consults with her gynecologist, who is unable to find objective evidence of a disease process but suggests that she cut back on work, relax more, and join an exercise class. Unfortunately, even though she drops down to a 20-hour work week, her symptoms continues to worsen. She is referred to a medical specialist who completes a full diagnostics workup, which suggests the diagnosis of chronic fatigue syndrome (CFS). Having a diagnosis provides Jennifer with a way to make sense of and explain her illness to others. Nevertheless, she experiences feelings of shame, self-hatred, and depression. She also feels increasingly isolated from her husband and coworkers. Her husband is increasingly upset with her "unavailability" and thinks he wants a divorce. Although her boss at the public defender's office is supportive, Jennifer fears that others will reject her, so she is very cautious in what she says to others. Unfortunately, this only makes the situation more complicated.

Phase 2

Jennifer's symptoms begin to stabilize, and she recognizes a pattern in her energy level and mood swings. She reads and talks widely to learn as much as she can about CFS, yet she is unable to find a health care professional who will guarantee a cure. There is growing conflict within her family and a loss of patience among some of her care providers. The persistence of her symptoms is increasingly frustrating for everyone. Her coworkers are annoyed that she is not keeping on top of her cases, and because she has reduced her hours even further, others are overwhelmed with attempting to represent many of her clients. Some have hinted that CFS is really a psychiatric disorder and that she should see a psychiatrist. She now knows what the word *stigma* really means, but she silently accepts this labeling and animus. However, she has developed a support system of two loyal friends, a nurse practitioner, and a psychotherapist whom she began seeing about her family, friend, and job concerns.

Phase 3

Jennifer is now experiencing longer periods of slight improvement and stability, which tends to be short lived and followed by relapses. She recognizes that efforts to return to being her old, productive self inevitably lead to relapse. As a result, she is less insistent on finding a cure and more on grieving the loss of her old self. With the help of the psychotherapist, she struggles to find a new sense of meaning in life and begins a daily diary. The prospect of a divorce and being on her own overwhelms her. Nevertheless, she is able to reach an amicable divorce agreement. Slowly, although painfully, a new self begins to emerge as she begins to consider and pursue new roles and new friends in her life. In time, she feels increasingly empowered and assertive in confronting others' bias and misinformation about CFS. Reducing her work commitment to 16 hours a week has been a godsend for her. This was made possible by the divorce stipulation that her former husband provide her full health insurance benefits.

Phase 4

Jennifer has become better at recognizing and accepting the waxing and waning course of her illness, and she now views relapse as inevitable but no longer as a failure. She has been able to incorporate some aspects of her pre-illness self into her newly emerging sense of self. Furthermore, she has also been able to reintegrate some of her formerly alienated family and friends. A college friend who had heard that she was divorced recently contacted her, and they have dated on a few occasions. Although it is too soon to say whether this relationship will deepen, Jennifer remains hopeful that her life has meaning and a purpose.

This case example accurately portrays how an individual with a chronic and debilitating condition like CFS can achieve a reasonably high level of wellness despite symptoms and change in social and occupational support. It also provides clinicians with a framework in which to establish treatment goals and plan interventions and anticipate resistance and clinician counter-transference (Fennell, 2003).

ISSUES UNIQUE TO CHRONIC ILLNESS

There are several clinical as well as theoretical issues that are associated with chronic illness. This section briefly reviews some of them.

Healing and Curing

Mind–body interventions frequently lead individuals to new ways of experiencing and expressing their illness. For instance, although *healing* usually denotes an objective improvement in health, individuals say they feel "healed" but not "cured." In other words, they experience a profound sense of overall well-being and wholeness even though the disease process is still present. Distinctions between *curing* (i.e., the actual eradication of a disease) and *healing* (i.e., a sense of wholeness) have little place in current medical practice but are, nevertheless, important. Because a cure is not common in chronic illness, acknowledging that healing without curing is a reality of life is essential in helping individuals accept and cope with their illness in a way that is both permissible and honorable (Fennell, 2003).

Health and Wellness

Wellness and *health care* are often used interchangeably, which is unfortunate because each term represents different, although related, realities. *Wellness* can be defined as "an integrated method of functioning, which is oriented toward maximizing the potential of which the individual is capable" (Dunn, 1961, p. 4). *Wellness* can also be viewed as a process of making choices for a successful existence (Hettler, 1984) or as "a way of life oriented toward an optimal state of health and well-being . . . that each individual is capable of achieving" (Myers, Sweeney, & Witmer, 2000, p. 252). Common to all three definitions is *choice* and *capability*, in which *capability* refers to the extent to which an optimal state of well-being is possible and achievable.

Pilch (1985) contended that both choice and capability are essential in understanding wellness. Furthermore, he distinguished *health* from *wellness* and envisions wellness as a continuum ranging from low to high that is parallel to health, which is also a continuum ranging from low to high. Accordingly, Pilch noted that individuals who are successful, conditioned athletes but use their strength to abuse and intimidate others might have achieved a high level of health but would be considered to have achieved only a low level of wellness. This is because such individuals have not chosen to "put their lives in proper perspective . . . to discover the true meaning of life" (p. 2). For Pilch, abusiveness would be incompatible with a wellness perspective wherein life is viewed as sacred.

Wellness is related to, but is independent of, health and health status. Wellness and health might be compared to two parallel sets of train tracks in which two trains, health and wellness, can move in the same or opposite directions, at the same speed or different speeds. My contention is that wellness is similar to health; wellness can coexist with chronic disease or even terminal illness. Thus, individuals can choose to experience a high level of wellness irrespective of their health status. The basic choice is to adopt or not to adopt a positive, life-giving attitude and endeavor to integrate or not integrate the past with the present. Individuals with high-level wellness may engage in preventive health behaviors, such as pursuing a healthy diet and exercising, to the extent to which they are able; such behaviors are not necessarily essential to wellness. Rather, wellness reflects individuals' life-affirming attitudes toward their bodies and others and the integration of these attitudes into their philosophy of life. Furthermore, the basic goal of all health counseling interventions is to improve health status and wellness, whichever the counselor is capable of achieving and to the degree that it is possible. Finally, capacity and choice are two key determinants of wellness. In short, wellness can coexist with chronic disease and even terminal illness, and individuals can experience a high level of wellness irrespective of their health status.

It is important to note that the concept of "wellness" itself rests within a set of cultural expectations and values. Considerable variation may exist between the concepts underlying Western ideas of wellness compared with the concepts underlying other traditional systems of healing. "American" culture, for example, has been viewed as overemphasizing the role of the individual at the expense of cultural, social, and political factors beyond an individual's control, which nonetheless strongly affect wellness (Bishop, 1998). Differing from an individualistic perspective, individuals with an Afrocentric worldview may believe that wellness and health springs from a harmony and balance with the natural order that comes from a connection and awareness with one's cultural heritage (Lewis, 2002).

In their quest to understand the phenomenon of illness, therapists need to be cognizant of the various wellness perspectives. Cultural factors influence biopsychosocial processes in the etiology; symptom manifestation and report; and diagnosis, assessment, intervention, and success of treatment outcomes (Mukherji, 1995). Traditional forms of wellness recognize that illness can influence one's sense of self and emphasize the holistic concept of healing. This holistic concept of health can extend beyond the individual to incorporate members of one's family and community. From this perspective, the health of an individual is virtually indistinguishable from the health of one's community (Garrett & Myers, 1996). If a culture or community is experiencing distress, members of that community or culture will invariably suffer. Therefore, across diagnosis and intervention, health counselors must continually be aware of the larger cultural context and social climate that surround individuals and their distress. From a therapeutic perspective, however, most interventions in the clinical realm will occur at the individual level.

Pain, Suffering, and Stigma

Pain and *suffering* are terms that are often used interchangeably as well as together, that is, *pain and suffering*. Although the terms are intimately related, they are quite different. *Pain* refers to the conscious experience of physical, emotional, or spiritual discomfort that is typically beyond the control of the individual. It may or may not hinder the individual's self-expression. However, *suffering* "goes beyond the conscious experience of discomfort. It includes certain knowledge of the influence of pain on one's life and an attitude of acceptance, indifference, or rejection with regard to the pain/discomfort" (Van der Poel, 1999, p. 35). Thus, suffering is essentially an individual's attitude toward his or her pain. Another way in which to think of the relationship between pain and suffering is that "suffering comes into existence when pain, even mild pain, persists and shows no indication of ever ending" (Fennell, 2003, p. 62).

For the most part, Americans attribute little if any positive value to suffering. Besides not really understanding it, they often regard it as frightening and meaningless. It is not surprising that in North America, the experience of the protracted pain associated with many chronic diseases lends itself to stigmatization. Seeing others suffer reminds most Americans that life is fragile, that individuals are easily hurt and disabled, and that they too will die or will experience similar suffering. Similarly, clinicians who encounter suffering in their work may, as Fennell (2003) stated,

> protect themselves against avoidance, anger, and despair by doing precisely what science advocates and the public desires. They locate a cause for the suffering as quickly as possible and provide appropriate treatment to end it. If, however, they cannot find the cause or if the suffering persists even with treatment, some clinicians become frustrated and even angry. Their personal fears begin to emerge [and they] may conclude that the suffering cannot have a physical genesis, but must proceed from psychological causes . . . [and the] implicit judgment of characterological failure, causing the sufferer to experience iatrogenic health care in the form of blame. (p. 63)

It is not surprising that individuals with chronic illness develop predictable responses to such attitudes. They consult a clinician in the hope of obtaining answers or at least solace but instead leave feeling confused, frightened, or blamed. As a result of such experiences, they may become more angry and sad and decide to avoid clinicians entirely. If they stay in treatment, they may avoid rejection by misrepresenting how they really feel and attempt to "pass" as healthy individuals. They may feel pressure to construct a public persona of "normalcy" to protect themselves from stigmatization. With its concomitant rejection of self and loss of self-esteem, such a dual existence "can lead to further avoidance of intimacy, increased isolation, substance abuse or alcoholism, martial problems, and sometimes suicide" (Fennell, 2003, p. 64).

Unfortunately, health care providers have limited knowledge of pain and suffering and tend to undertreat pain because of this lack of knowledge or because of inadequate assessment (Erlen, 2002). The challenge for health care providers is to expand their perspective and treatment repertoire. They must come to view pain and suffering as more than simply unpleasant sensations to be managed by medication, surgery, or distraction techniques. They need to recognize and acknowledge the limitation of conventional pain management protocols and strive to more adequately address the attitudinal dimension of pain, that is, suffering, which is more likely to respond to spiritual or psychotherapeutic interventions.

Spiritual and Religious Issues in Chronic Illness

The experience of chronic illness often engenders a religious or evidential crisis, or at least a reconsideration of core values and beliefs, for most individuals. The nature of this crisis or reconsideration is dependent largely on cultural factors and religious upbringing, and its urgency tends to be driven by the extent to which the disease is life threatening or disability provoking. The nature and expression of these spiritual issues varies by phase of the illness (Fennell, 2003).

Phase 1

The urgency and lack of control that is experienced over individuals' physical and psychological well-being can manifest in a rather primitive manner. As Fennell (2003) discussed, to the extent to which they

> believe they are bad for being ill and yet cannot in any fashion change the facts of their situation or fix themselves, they tend to believe either that God has abandoned them, or that there is no God at all, or that God is punishing them. (pp. 174–175)

Many Westerners who believe in a deity imagine that deity as an angry and avenging God who levies bad fortune—particularly under the guise of illness—as a sign of deserved punishment. However, those who are atheists may experience deep existential dread and despair and conclude that they have no reason to continue living because there is no longer any point in living. The end result is deep grief for such believers and nonbelievers.

Phase 2

In this phase, those who are believers may no longer conclude that God is punishing them, but rather that God has turned his attention away from them. It is not surprising that the experience of chronic illness draws many back to religious or spiritual practices, often if their religious affiliation is highly structured and hierarchical. They, as Fennell (2003) noted, "often believe that they will return to their former state of health if they perform prayers and practice rituals sincerely, properly, and over a long enough period of time . . . that God will eventually reward their compliant behavior" (p. 248) However, others may reject the God of their past and seek more satisfying spiritual meaning and connections with like-minded individuals and settings in which they are treated empathically and their suffering is understood.

Phase 3

Of all the phases, Phase 3 involves the most serious spiritual undertaking. In this phase, individuals with a chronic disease search for an explanation for their illness, even though that explanation may be that it occurred randomly and without any divine or other intention. They "need to generate for themselves a genuine sense of purpose—not simply some traditional bromide foisted off on those the society regards as damaged, but something the patient can sincerely and personally commit to" (Fennell, 2003, p. 304). In this phase, they become committed to truth and authenticity as they undertake to construct a new self, a self that reflects their experience of chronicity. It is not surprising that when the tenets of their prior religious beliefs seem inauthentic or inadequate to their new conception self, they seek out new spiritual resources and affiliations.

Phase 4

In this phase, individuals move beyond the search for a sense of meaning of Phase 3 to a search to find meaning in all their relationships and all their daily activities:

> Now it is not the practiced value of an activity that concerns them, but rather its overall place and meaning in their existence. Their heightened awareness makes patients demand more from everything they do. They may have to live with pain and limitations, but they can insist that whatever they do will be meaningful. (Fennell, 2003, pp. 341–342)

METHODS AND APPROACHES FOR TREATING CHRONIC ILLNESS

Were it simply a matter of providing individuals who are chronically ill with health-related information about lifestyle change, the clinical task would be relatively simple. Although health information is necessary, it is seldom sufficient to achieve health behavior change (Jordan-Marsh, Gilbert, Ford, & Kleeman, 1984). Helping individuals achieve health behavior change requires an understanding of the barriers to change and the requisite counseling and psychotherapy strategies and skills to accomplish such change. This section first describes different methods for effecting change and then comments on the use of various psychotherapeutic approaches with chronic illness.

Methods for Effecting Health Behavior Change

Five methods for effecting health behavior change can be described. Table 1.1 summarizes the focus, strategies, and typical provider or facilitator of change. For a fuller discussion of these approaches, the reader is referred to Sperry, Lewis, Carlson, and Englar-Carlson (2005).

Medical Care Counseling

Physicians typically broach the health matter, ask a few questions, give focused information, and prescribe some behavior change, all within a very

TABLE 1.1
Health Change Methods

Method	Focus, strategies, and typical provider
Medical care counseling	Improve compliance with a treatment regimen; primarily, a provider-centered intervention wherein treatment is prescribed and the patient is expected to follow it; usually involves a minimal degree of education and monitoring. Usually provided by physicians.
Patient care counseling	Improve patient capacity for self-management; usually involves some degree of collaboration and focuses on understanding, skill mastery, and self-monitoring of symptoms and regimen; involves individual and group educational methods. Usually provided by nurses, dieticians, and patient educators.
Health promotion counseling	Improve lifestyle, health behaviors, and health status in light of psychological principles—assessment, establishing a collaborative relationship with patients, interventions tailored to needs and expectations, and relapse prevention. Usually provided by health counselors and nurse practitioners.
Health-focused counseling	Improve lifestyle, health behaviors, and health status by increasing adherence to a health prescription when barriers are present or anticipated—assessment of needs, strengths, and readiness; engage in the treatment process; focus on tailored interventions and relapse prevention; and use cognitive restructuring and other strategies to reduce barriers to change. Usually provided by primary care physicians and other health care providers with some formal counseling training or by psychotherapists.
Health-focused psychotherapy	Improve health status in difficult and complex case in which acceptance of life-threatening, severely impairing, or progressively debilitating illness, intractable pain, and so on, is difficult; significant personality and systemic dynamics complicate the treatment process; psychotherapeutic strategies and tactics to modify maladaptive schemas and family narratives, that is, schema therapy, interpretation, and so on. Provided by psychotherapists with specialized training in treating chronic illness.

short time frame. Usually, patients are given the prescription to change behaviors, that is, lose weight, stop smoking, or take up exercise. The goal of this approach is to improve health status by implementing the health prescription or recommendation. Change or improvement is assumed to occur because the patient follows the provider's health prescription. This approach also assumes that patients comply with the health prescriptions because of their confidence and belief in the providers' expertise and authority. Typically, this type of counseling involves some limited advisement as to the need for the change and some general guidelines to follow. Usually, there is a minimal degree of education and monitoring. If the patient is not able to follow this advice, for whatever reason, referral may be made for "patient education," or what I refer to in this book as *patient care counseling.*

Patient Care Counseling

Patient care counseling—also called *patient education* and *psycho-education*, and sometimes *self-management*—is typically provided by physician extenders, such as nurses, nurse practitioners, or patient educators. Its purpose is to improve patient understanding, skill, and compliance with health prescriptions and, most important, to foster the individual's capacity to engage in self-management. Self-management requires a repertoire of health-oriented skills, a belief in one's own ability to address life's challenges, and an environment that encourages positive development. In addition, it provides support as well as the technical assistance necessary to help individuals carry out their choices. It is assumed that prescribed change occurs because the patient sufficiently understands and has adequately practiced or mastered the prescribed change regimen. Assessment typically involves estimating the patient's understanding of the need for treatment, the treatment regimen, and the degree of mastery of any requisite skills necessary for compliance with the regimen. A variety of intervention strategies are used. These include individual or group educational methods. Monitoring compliance is essential for successful patient care counseling. Compared with medical care counseling, there is considerably more assessment, education, and monitoring in patient care counseling.

Health Promotion Counseling

Quite different from both the physician and the physician extender, the health promotion specialist usually begins with a general screening assessment, such as a formal health risk appraisal instrument. The individual being assessed may not see him- or herself in the patient role or present with signs or symptoms of disease. At its best, this approach to health counseling is tailored to the individual's needs and expectations. It may also identify the individual's level of readiness for change and barriers to adherence to lifestyle change. The primary goal of this approach is to improve lifestyle and health behaviors. It is assumed that change occurs because of the collaboration in the process of establishing, practicing, and monitoring a tailored health promotion intervention. Because personal skills are so crucial, health promotion counseling uses educational methods aimed toward skill building. Relapse prevention is increasingly a component in successful health promotion endeavors. Also, because a sense of control is associated with positive clinical outcomes, this approach uses interventions designed to increase one's perceptions of control and self-efficacy.

Health-Focused Counseling

Patients referred for this method have been unsuccessful in patient care or health promotion counseling, usually because of compliance issues due to internal or external barriers. The goal of this approach is to reduce symptoms and improve health status, to improve lifestyle and positive health behaviors, or to increase adherence to a health prescription. It is assumed that change occurs because the patient is sufficiently engaged in and collaborates with the tailored intervention process and because barriers to change, that is, intrapersonal, interpersonal, social, and cultural barriers, are recognized and dealt with. Effective use of this method requires that the patient's readiness for change be sufficient before proceeding with the prescribed change effort. Accordingly, providers must have some proficiency in using motivational counseling strategies to promote readiness (Miller & Rollnick, 2002). Assessment typically includes an evaluation of maladaptive beliefs and thinking errors, readiness for change, strengths, and barriers—psychological, relational, situational, and cultural—that have impeded, or could have impeded, adherence to a change program. Tailored interventions and relapse prevention are core treatment strategies. Several psychotherapeutic interventions, such as reframing and cognitive restructuring, as well as other systemic strategies, are used to reduce barriers to change. It is not surprising that CBT approaches that have been adapted to chronic illness (C. A. White, 2001) are particularly consistent with health-focused counseling. Psychotherapists— that is, social workers, psychologists, marital and family therapists, mental health counselors, and psychiatrists, as well as primary care physicians and nurse practitioners—can and do provide such health-focused counseling.

Health-Focused Psychotherapy

Individuals referred for this approach tend to have experienced significant difficulty with acceptance of their illness or its impairment, coping with a rapidly progressing, severely debilitating, or life-threatening condition, managing intractable pain, and so on. In many instances, their illness dynamics overlap considerably with their personality dynamics and family systems dynamics. Such biopsychosocial complexity and severity are the principal indicators for the use of health-focused psychotherapy instead of health-focused counseling (Sperry et al., 2005). There are obvious similarities between conventional psychotherapy and health-focused psychotherapy; however, there are some differences. Chief among these is the emphasis placed on a comprehensive assessment of the individual, particularly the impact of the disease process on the individual, as well as the influence of personality and family dynamics on the illness. Rather than using interventions that modify thinking errors and maladaptive beliefs as in health-focused counseling, health-focused psychotherapy interventions are used that modify core personality dynamics—that is, maladaptive schemas—and family dynamics are the mainstays that tend to be used. This approach is best provided by psychotherapists with specialized knowledge, skills, and experience in treating chronic illness. For those operating from a CBT perspective, skill and experience in using schema-focused therapy (Young, Klosko, & Weishaar,

2003) are consistent with what we are describing as health-focused psycho-therapy, as are many of the brief dynamic psychotherapy approaches (Binder, 2004).

Distinguishing Health-Focused Counseling From Health-Focused Psychotherapy

Why is a distinction being made between *health-focused counseling* and *health-focused psychotherapy*? Are they not really the same? The distinction is necessary because of the severity and complexity of the cases, practice patterns and practice sites, and research protocols. First and foremost, health-focused psychotherapy is indicated in difficult, complex, and so-called treatment-resistant cases. However, health-focused counseling is indicated for cases of low to moderate difficulty. Second is the matter of practice patterns and practice sites. The reality is that physicians and nurse practitioners, as well as others with very limited psychotherapy training and experience, provide a considerable amount of what I am calling *health-focused counseling*, particularly in primary care settings. Although some licensed psychotherapists do work in primary care medical settings, the majority work in what research protocols refer to as *secondary care settings*. *Primary care* refers to settings that emphasize primary or general care provided by generalists, whereas *secondary care* refers to settings that emphasize specialized care provided by specialists. I would consider a licensed psychotherapist to be a specialist. When nonspecialists, such as primary care physicians, are trained to provide cognitive–behavioral treatment of chronic illness, they are taught to use a few very basic CBT methods, for example, self-monitoring, experimentation, and changing distressing automatic thoughts (Sadovsky, 2002). Using a few such CBT methods does not mean the physician is providing cognitive–behaviorally oriented psychotherapy. Third, as detailed in a subsequent section, research studies, particularly meta-analyses of several CBT studies, show significant differences between CBT practiced in primary care settings and that practiced in secondary care settings.

Psychotherapeutic Approaches to Chronic Illness

Of the various psychotherapy systems and approaches used in both primary care and secondary care settings, three are commonly used in treating chronic illness: brief psychodynamic therapy, CBT, and hypnotherapy. The application of each of these approaches to the treatment of irritable bowel syndrome (IBS)—a very common chronic illness—is briefly described here.

Brief Psychodynamic Therapy

Brief psychodynamic therapy with IBS is conducted in an individual format once a week for 2 to 3 months. The goal is to explore and identify potential unconscious factors that may be linked to IBS symptoms and to achieve insight and control by bringing those factors into consciousness. Because buried feelings cause emotional distress that in turn triggers bowel symptoms, this therapy helps individuals to consciously realize that resentment toward others underlies their symptoms. It then provides various strategies for coping with feelings. Strategies might include confronting the offending person or refusing to become involved in situations that make the individual feel bad.

Cognitive Therapy and Cognitive–Behavioral Therapy

CBT with IBS is conducted in an individual or group format. The premise is that patients with IBS hold maladaptive beliefs and engage in negative automatic thinking. For instance, individuals might routinely assume more responsibility for situations, believing if they do not do it, it will not be done right, or they may catastrophize about such situations, thinking they will not meet a deadline and so will be fired. In this approach, the patient is asked to monitor his or her bowel symptoms and thoughts and feelings associated with them. Therapists explain how conscious negative messages cause stress and subsequent bowel symptoms, and they help individuals to identify negative beliefs, thoughts, and self-talk, as well as ways of replacing them with more realistic positive thoughts and self-talk. Subsequent sessions enable individuals to gradually react more positively to stressors, which translates into reduced bowel symptoms.

Hypnotherapy

Hypnotherapy with IBS can be conducted in either an individual or a group format. It uses imagery to gain control over the muscles of the gut and bowel. The therapist induces a light trance, that is, a focused, calm, and relaxed state, and then encourages patients to imagine their bowel muscles as very smooth and calm. Those who successfully make use of the imagery report less pain, bloating, cramping, diarrhea, and constipation. Such imagery can be combined with cognitive–behavioral strategies to affect increased treatment outcomes.

Research on Psychotherapeutic Treatment of Irritable Bowel Syndrome

Researchers have compared the effectiveness of brief psychodynamic psychotherapy, hypnotherapy, CBT, and cognitive therapy in the treatment of IBS. Blanchard and Malamood's (1996) analysis of studies before 1995 indicated that each of these treatment approaches was superior to symptom monitoring or routine medical care, although cognitive therapy and hypnotherapy were found to be superior to placebo control conditions. It is interesting to note that these outcomes were maintained up to 4 years (Blanchard & Malamood, 1996). A more recent review of studies of treatments of IBS in adults and its likely developmental precursor in children, recurrent abdominal pain (RAP), further supported the efficacy of hypnotherapy, cognitive therapy, and brief psychodynamic psychotherapy for IBS. It was also found that CBT that combines operant elements and stress management was most effective in the treatment of RAP (Blanchard & Scharff, 2002).

Cognitive–Behavioral Therapy and Cognitive–Behavioral Treatment of Chronic Illness

CBT and cognitive–behavioral treatment are the most commonly practiced, as well as most commonly researched, treatment approaches with chronic illness in both primary and secondary care settings. It is important to distinguish between these two. *CBT* refers to a coherent and structured approach to assessment, case conceptualization, intervention, and relapse prevention on the basis of cognitive and behavioral principles and philosophy of treatment, in other words, the essential elements of CBT. However, *cognitive–behavioral treatments* refers to the use of cognitive or behavioral treatment strategies without the coherence, structure, or philosophy of treatment underlying CBT. Unfortunately, many self-management protocols and programs use such cognitive–behavioral treatments in the form of skill-training activities, monitoring and modifying automatic negative thoughts, homework assignments, and so on, but label them as CBT programs. Although cognitive–behavioral treatments, also called *cognitive–behavioral counseling* (C. A. White, 2001), can be effective interventions, they are not technically CBT and should not be designated as such. Although this distinction may not be critical in the clinical realm, it is critical in the research realms, as is noted later in this chapter. This section describes both training materials and research on the effectiveness of CBT in the treatment of chronic illness.

Training Materials

An Internet search of CBT and various chronic diseases yields an incredible list of both clinically focused articles and book chapters, not to mention empirical studies. Publishing trends show the number of book chapters and books on cognitive therapy, behavior therapy, and CBT treatment of chronic illness has expanded greatly since 2000, and there is every indication that this trend will continue. Currently, there are at least two CBT books directed at professionals that address the general treatment of chronic medical illnesses (Sharoff, 2004; C. A. White, 2001). In addition, there are several CBT books that focus on specific chronic medical illnesses. These include chronic pain (Eimer & Freeman, 1999; Thorn, 2004; Winterowd, Beck, & Gruener, 2004), cancer (Moorey & Greer, 2003), IBS (Segal, Toner, Emmott, & Myran, 2000), and AIDS (Crawford & Fishman, 1997).

Empirical Research

Several studies have been reported on the effectiveness of CBT with specific chronic illnesses. Looking just at Type 1 diabetes, also called *juve-*

nile-onset diabetes because it presents in childhood and usually is much more severe than Type 2 diabetes, research suggests that CBT can be a particularly effective intervention. One study looked at a CBT group treatment of individuals with Type 1 diabetes and a history of poor glycemic control and found that CBT was effective in improving glycemic control (Snoek, van der Ven, & Lubach, 1999). Another study showed that time-limited CBT interventions decreased the severity of psychological problems, that is, depression and anxiety, and improved glycemic control in Type 1 adult diabetic patients with microvascular complications (Didjurgeit, Kruse, Schmitz, Stuckenschneider, & Sawicki, 2002). These are just two of several dozens of studies on CBT and diabetes. In comparison, I found only one study on psychodynamic treatment of Type 1 diabetes. In this study of children with diabetes with very poor glycemic control who required repeated hospital admissions, when offered intensive inpatient psychoanalytic psychotherapy three to four times a week for an average of 15 weeks, they achieved significant glycemic control that was maintained for at least 1 year, compared with an equivalent group (Moran, Fonagy, Kurtz, Bolton, & Brook, 1991).

Meta-Analyses

Large meta-analyses have proved valuable in comparing psychotherapy approaches. In a recently reported study (Raine et al., 2002) involving psychological treatments of chronic illness, several findings are noteworthy. The results of meta-analyses and of randomized controlled trials of 61 studies indicated that CBT and behavior therapy were particularly effective for chronic back pain and chronic fatigue syndrome but were not as effective as antidepressants for IBS. CBT and behavior therapy were also noted to be more effective in situations in which these conditions were treated in secondary care settings by specialists, that is, psychotherapists, rather than by primary care providers. Presumably, individuals referred to these therapists presented with more complex symptoms and circumstances than those who were treated in primary care settings and did not need a referral. Accordingly, this meta-analysis suggests that specialized training in CBT and behavior therapy can make a difference in effectively treating individuals with complex or difficult or chronic illness presentations (Raine et al., 2002). These researchers indicated that some studies they reviewed appeared to involve cognitive–behavioral treatment rather than formal CBT. Presumably, it was provided by nonpsychotherapists in primary care settings, whereas CBT was more likely to be provided by psychotherapists in secondary care settings. Besides distinguishing between the providers and settings, this meta-analytic study raised the following considerations. One was that the level of training and expertise of the providers appeared to account for differential outcomes. A second was that patient readiness and engagement in the treatment process may have impacted outcomes. A third was that providing cognitive–behavioral treatment has limitations and that providing a focal type of CBT may be preferable. Although not discussed in this meta-analysis study, it seems that providing conventional CBT to patients with chronic illness is probably less effective than CBT that is tailored to the treatment of chronic illness. Presumably, this is due in part to assessment. Assessment in conventional CBT emphasizes eliciting negative automatic thinking, intermediate beliefs, and core beliefs, although assessment in CBT directed at chronic illness emphasizes eliciting the patient's perception of his or her illness and tailoring treatment accordingly (C. A. White, 2001).

BIOPSYCHOSOCIAL THERAPY: A BRIEF GLIMPSE

This book describes a clinical approach to chronic illness called Biopsychosocial Therapy that is broad and inclusive and is particularly compatible with CBT. This Biopsychosocial Therapy approach is a health-focused psychotherapy method indicated primarily for difficult and complex cases. Whereas chapter 5 describes Biopsychosocial Therapy in detail, this section briefly points out some of its unique features in treating chronic illness. One of those features is assessment.

The assessment strategy in the biopsychosocial treatment of chronic illnesses is unique. In traditional and conventional psychotherapy, the assessment is focused primarily on psychological and psychosocial factors. Like most effective psychotherapy approaches, the Biopsychosocial Therapy approach to chronic illness identifies key psychological factors along with cogent social, family, and cultural factors. In addition, the Biopsychosocial Therapy approach identifies other critical information, such as the level of disease progression, the degree of impairment, symptoms and their triggers, the meaning of the illness, and the explanation the patient has for that illness, along with his or her inner and outer resources. Such a comprehensive assessment permits us to plan a psychotherapeutic intervention that is informed by the biological dimension as well as by the psychosocial and cultural dimensions.

Biopsychosocial Therapy begins by engaging the individual with the chronic illness in the treatment process. The therapist begins by listening attentively, responding empathically, and establishing a therapeutic relationship. As this is developing, the therapist works to elicit a rather complete biopsychosocial assessment that leads to the development of a biopsychosocial case conceptualization. Because this case conceptualization is central to choosing, sequencing, and implementing effective interventions, it is essential that the biopsychosocial assessment be comprehensive and complete. Because chronic illnesses are biopsychosocial entities, effective treatment of difficult, complex, or treatment-resistant cases requires a biopsychosocial perspective and multifaceted biopsychosocial interventions.

CONCLUDING NOTE

Although *chronic disease* is largely an objective entity, *chronic illness* is the subjective experience of a chronic disease. As individuals live longer, the incidence and prevalence of chronic disease will increase and, along with it, the expectation—of those experiencing such illness—to maintain the highest quality of life possible. The challenge is for health care providers, particularly psychotherapists, to provide effective health-focused counseling and psychotherapy to ameliorate symptoms, minimize disease progression, and increase wellness. Health-focused counseling and health-focused psychotherapy were described and differentiated, and Biopsychosocial Therapy was briefly introduced. Practicing effective health-focused counseling and health-focused psychotherapy requires some specialized knowledge, skills, and experience. This book endeavors to provide some of the knowledge and skill base needed for providing such interventions to individuals, particularly those with challenging and difficult-to-treat chronic illness.

2

BIOPSYCHOSOCIAL MODEL
OF CHRONIC ILLNESS

This book is about the biopsychosocial approach to treating chronic illness. But what exactly is the biopsychosocial model, and how does it differ from the psychological or psychosocial model that is more familiar to psychologists and other mental health professionals? Why is this biopsychosocial model germane in working with patients with chronic illnesses?

This chapter addresses these and other related questions. It begins with a discussion of the need for and value of the biopsychosocial model. Then it describes this model and contrasts it with the biomedical model and psychosocial model of illness. In this book, the social dimension of the biopsychosocial model is a shorthand designation for the sociocultural dimension. Because cultural factors significantly influence the context and the way in which chronic illness is understood and experienced and the way in which individuals respond to providers and the treatment process, relevant cultural aspects of chronic illness are discussed. Another social dimension is family dynamics and the way in which these dynamics impact and are impacted by chronic illness. This important topic is also considered. Finally, a case study illustrates many of the concepts of this chapter, including family dynamics.

[handwritten margin note: not psych or psych/ social]

[handwritten margin note: definitions of model]

25

NEED FOR THE BIOPSYCHOSOCIAL MODEL AND PERSPECTIVE

Health care in the United States is in a critical state today and has little likelihood of being resuscitated without a critical reexamination of some of its basic premises. One of these basic premises is that mind and body are separate. The result of such dualistic thinking is the supremacy of the biomedical model in health care. Although this model has been championed by the medical profession, the psychology profession has until recently subscribed to a psychological model or psychosocial model of health:

> By maintaining the fiction that mind and body are separate, and further, assuming that the only role that the mind plays in health and illness is in mental health and illness, we have developed a healthcare system that is hobbled it its ability to deal with the many varied roles that mind and behavior play in so-called physical illness. (Levant, 2004, p. 8)

The reality is, however, that behavioral factors are intimately related to health status and disease conditions. For instance, the nation's leading causes of death are largely the result of health-damaging behaviors such as obesity, tobacco use, alcohol abuse, injuries, suicide, and unprotected sex (Centers for Disease Control and Prevention, 2002). Another way of conceptualizing the enormity of the problem is that an estimated 40% of deaths annually are attributable to modifiable behaviors (McGinnis, Williams-Russo, & Knickman, 2002). Unfortunately, neither the biomedical model nor the psychological model is sufficient to explain, treat, or prevent what are essentially biopsychosocial illnesses. In short, a biopsychosocial model and treatment perspective is needed to inform assessment, diagnosis, treatment, and prevention. In the medical profession, the specialties of psychiatry and family medicine have embraced the biopsychosocial model for about 30 years, although pediatrics and internal medicine have more recently begun to incorporate it into training and clinical practice. Other specialties, particularly the surgical subspecialties, have been much slower to adopt this model.

Psychology as a profession is at the brink of major change with regard to the biopsychosocial model. One of the first indications of a shift from the psychological model to the biopsychosocial model has been a recent change in the identity of psychology from that of a mental health profession to a health profession with mental health as an area of expertise. Since 2001, the American Psychological Association's mission statement has included promoting health as part of its mission. It is not surprising that this change in identity and mission necessitates a shift in perspective from the psychological model and psychosocial perspective to a biopsychosocial model and perspective. Levant (2004) noted that "viewing psychology as a health discipline operating from a biopsychosocial perspective will require, of course, a dramatic change" (p. 10). Although he was referring largely to dramatic changes in graduate training programs, changes in clinician attitudes and practice patterns will also require radical restructuring.

WHAT IS THE BIOPSYCHOSOCIAL MODEL?

The biopsychosocial model is a comprehensive and systemic perspective for understanding the person and the relationship of the system outside and inside the person that influences both health and illness (Engel, 1977; Nicassio & Smith, 1995; Sperry, 1988). Unlike the biomedical model, which views the cause of an illness in terms of linear thinking—that is, diseases have a single cause and usually a single treatment—the biopsychosocial model described in this chapter views illness in terms of general systems theory or systemic thinking. In systemic thinking, a web of interactions of several factors, rather than a single factor, "causes" an illness. Health is sustained by a state of balance among a web of factors: biological, psychological, social, environmental, and so on.

The biopsychosocial model proposes that a person can be adequately understood only if the therapist considers all levels of the person's functioning: biological, psychological, and social. *Biological functioning* refers to all peripheral organ system functions, as well as to all autonomic, neuroendocrine, and central nervous system functions that are subcortical—that is, to all processes that are automatic and outside conscious awareness. *Psychological functioning* refers to the self-conscious inner world that directs information processing and communication from and with the outside world. It basically involves cortical structures and conscious awareness. It also includes the internal representation of self, the world, and personal goals, which reflects aspirations, ideals, needs, and the cognitions and strategies that govern behavior. *Social functioning* refers to the person's behavior in relation to family, friends, authorities, peer group, and cultural expectations, as well as community institutions that influence and are influenced by the individual. It may well be that a fully comprehensive biopsychosocial approach would also include the spiritual or life-meaning dimension of functioning (Sperry, 2003a).

FROM THE BIOMEDICAL AND PSYCHOSOCIAL MODELS TO THE BIOPSYCHOSOCIAL MODEL

The biopsychosocial model has evolved from dissatisfaction with both the biomedical and psychosocial models of health and illness. It is useful to understand some of the theoretical and research basis for the biomedical and psychosocial models to appreciate the theoretical contribution and clinical utility of the biopsychosocial model. In this section, I briefly review the biomedical, the psychosocial, and the biopsychosocial models and highlight their commonalities and differences. I also illustrate each of these models with a chronic disease, rheumatoid arthritis (RA). RA is a serious chronic illness that well exemplifies the biopsychosocial model because it involves obvious pathophysiological factors as well as significant psychosocial factors.

Biomedical Model

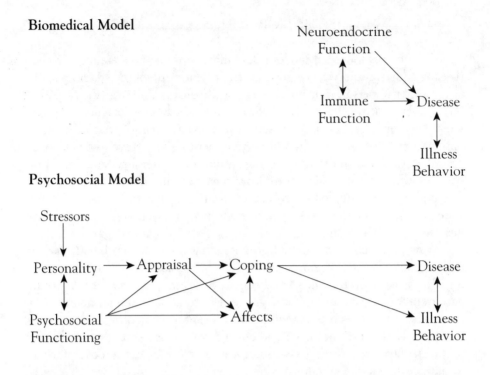

Psychosocial Model

Biopsychosocial Model

Figure 2.1. Three models of the pathogenesis of rheumatoid arthritis. Data from Walker, Jackson, and Littlejohn (2004).

Figure 2.1 summaries this discussion with a visual representation of each of the three models.

Biomedical Model

The biomedical model focuses on disease and disability—their causes, prevention, and cure—and is the most widely used conceptualization of disease processes in medical research. RA is a chronic inflammatory rheumatic disease that targets the synovial lining of the joints, bursae, and tendon

sheaths, which when inflamed, results in synovitis and the erosion of cartilage and bone. In time, destruction of the joint occurs. RA is believed to be
caused by multiple factors, including genetic predispositions, environmental
factors, and, particularly, immune and neuroendocrine functions. A biomedical model of RA is rendered in Figure 2.1 and emphasizes the immune and
neuroendocrine functions. Although this diagram is somewhat simplified and
probably includes other feedback loops, it is a useful summary of the pathways and interactions involved.

bio-medical

A number of criticisms of the limitations of the biomedical model of
illness can be made. First and foremost, it does not account for the complexity of psychological, social, and environmental factors involved in the illness
process. Some have suggested that psychosocial and environmental factors
play a significant role in both the etiology and progression of a number of
chronic illnesses that the biomedical model underplays (Cioffi, 1991). Another thorny issue with this model is that someone can report being ill without obvious pathophysiology. Particularly perplexing is the situation of an
individual who has been diagnosed with a chronic condition like RA but
experiences few, if any, symptoms, pain, or disability (Chamie, 1995). In
short, the biomedical model assumes that there is a linear one-to-one relationship among pathophysiology, disease progression, and disability.

Why does the biomedical model continue to be dominant today? There
are several reasons. Briefly, physicians' training and experience predispose
them to view patients' signs and symptoms from this model and to underplay
patients' complaints related to psychosocial factors. Because their professional
identities are based on a biomedical viewpoint, and because practice patterns
and diagnostic codes emphasize physical diagnosis, there is little incentive to
focus on psychosocial factors that are the domain of other providers, that is,
psychologists and counselors. Existing payment mechanisms also favor physical
diagnosis and treatment that further reinforce adherence to the biomedical
model. It is also interesting to note that the biomedical model is reinforced
by patients who present only physical complaints that they attribute to a
physical cause. Essentially, they collude with their physician's selective focus
on the biomedical factors, rather than on psychological symptoms and psychosocial causes (Zimmerman & Tansella, 1996).

why bio-medical

Psychosocial Model

psycho-social

Coping with stressors, such as chronic illness, continues to be a mainstay of psychological research. Lazarus and Folkman's (1984) stress and coping paradigm has been used extensively in research as a way of understanding
the role of psychological and psychosocial processes in chronic illness. In
this paradigm, *coping* refers to cognitive and behavioral responses to events
perceived as taxing or harmful to an individual's well-being (Lazarus &
Folkman, 1984). Several distinct components of the coping process have

been identified, notably appraisals of harm or threat to self-worth posed by a stressor and the degree of controllability of the outcome and recurrence of the stressful situation (Zautra & Manne, 1992). Assuming that individuals are constantly appraising their relationship to the environment, the stress process begins with an appraisal of an actual or threatened change and an evaluation of its personal significance. This is called a *primary appraisal*, and the evaluation of the options for coping is referred to as *secondary appraisal*. *Primary appraisal* includes the appraisals of harm or loss that have already occurred, threatened harm or loss, or challenge—referring to the opportunity for mastery or gain—and is influenced by an individual's beliefs (Folkman & Greer, 2000). Thus, appraisals of an event, such as the diagnosis of a rheumatic condition, will be assessed differently because individuals differ in these attributes. *Secondary appraisal* involves the extent to which the situation is one that can be controlled or changed by the individual, such as feelings of helplessness and locus of control. Such beliefs are critical in the secondary appraisal of changeability or options for controlling the situation. The best known of these beliefs is self-efficacy (Bandura, 1997), which includes *outcome efficacy*, that is, the belief that there is a strategy that will result in the desired outcome, and *self-efficacy*, that is, the belief that the individual can use that strategy to achieve the outcome.

An individual's characteristics, such as personality traits—particularly optimism, neuroticism, and hardiness—are believed to influence, for better or worse, his or her ability to appraise situations realistically, to choose the appropriate coping strategy, and to use it effectively (Folkman & Greer, 2000). Thus, personality characteristics, such as optimism, can influence an individual's appraisal of the threat posed by illness or daily minor stressors, as well as the capacity to deal with those stressors, which can either exacerbate or reduce RA symptoms and disease progression. Such appraisals also influence the coping strategies used, which may lead to changes in affect, which can impact disease activity, as well as specific illness behaviors such as pain levels, disability, and medication use. Unlike the biomedical model, the psychosocial model assumes that, rather than being linear, the interface between psychosocial and biological variables is complex, with dynamic and reciprocal associations. Accordingly, pain and disability can be conceptualized as significant predictors of psychological well-being (Hagglund, Halley, Reveille, & Alacren, 1989).

Biopsychosocial Model

The biopsychosocial model offers a broader and more integrative perspective than the biomedical and psychosocial models. A promising framework for conceptualizing the relationship between biological and psychosocial factors in chronic illness is a vulnerability model wherein minor chronic stressors can promote disease progression (Zautra, Burleson, Matt, Roth, &

Burrows, 1994). In other words, a sufficient amount of additional daily stressors can precipitate an illness episode. In this model, the interaction among stressors, coping efficacy, and neuroendocrine function affect disease status (Zautra et al., 1994). An integrated biopsychosocial model has recently been proposed that accounts for the effect of stressors, personality, psychosocial functioning, and coping efficacy, as well as immune and neuroendocrine function, on disease progression and illness behavior in RA (Walker, Jackson, & Littlejohn, 2004).

This integrated biopsychosocial model is based on an expanded version of the stress and coping paradigm (Monat & Lazarus, 1991) and provides a convincing operational definition of the biopsychosocial approach (Zimmerman & Tansella, 1996). In the expanded paradigm, stress is conceptualized as incorporating psychological, physiological, and environmental levels as well as including elements such as daily hassles, the perception of an event as threatening, distressed affect, and associated changes in neuroendocrine functioning (Monat & Lazarus, 1991).

In the integrated biopsychosocial model, psychosocial stressors influence RA disease activity not directly, but rather indirectly, through a cycle of psychosocial responses that either reduce or exacerbate the effects of the psychosocial stressor on the RA condition:

> Cognitive appraisals of the threat posed by the stressor and available resources play a central role in the impact of stressors on psychosocial and physical outcomes. None of these processes are considered to be linear but rather involve cycles and feedback loops over time. (Walker et al., 2004, p. 481)

In short, such a biopsychosocial model of chronic illness based on an expanded stress and coping paradigm that incorporates aspects of psychosocial functioning, personality, and immune and neuroendocirine functioning offers a comprehensive approach to assessing and treating rheumatic conditions and may be heuristic in conceptualizing other chronic illness processes as well (Walker et al., 2004).

BIOPSYCHOSOCIAL DIMENSIONS OF STRESS

The biopsychosocial model described in the previous section possesses a certain elegance. It not only integrates a number of key constructs and theories from the biological and psychological sciences, but it also provides a succinct "map" of the process of disease development and progression—that is, *pathogenesis*—which allows "entry points" or leverage for both treatment and prevention interventions. A perusal of the biopsychosocial model map in Figure 2.1 reveals a complex web of linkages between two key variables: stress and disease. Stress, primarily psychological stress, has long been a key construct in understanding psychopathology. Recently, stress has become a key construct for understanding the pathogenesis of chronic disease. This stress is referred to in the medical literature as *oxidative stress*.

Stress and Oxidative Stress

Even though the average life expectancy in North America has increased dramatically during this past century, quality of life has actually decreased because of chronic illness. The incidence of coronary artery disease, cancer, diabetes, Alzheimer's disease, Parkinson's disease, arthritis, and macular degeneration continues to increase as oxidative stress increases. Oxidative stress is widely recognized as the underlying cause of chronic disease as well as of aging (Lane, 2003). What exactly is oxidative stress, and what, if any, relationship does it have to psychological stress?

Within every cell of the body are mitochondria that serve an energy-producing function that can be likened to that of a furnace. As oxygen is used within this cellular furnace to create energy, a charged oxygen molecule—called a *free radical*—is occasionally produced. Free radicals have an unpaired electron in their outer orbit, giving them an electrical charge. If a free radical is not readily neutralized by an antioxidant, it can create more volatile free radicals that damage cell walls, vessel walls, proteins, fats, and even DNA.

Free-radical activity is not necessarily harmful. Without free-radical activity, cells would be unable to produce energy, maintain immunity, transmit nerve impulses, synthesize hormones, or even contract muscles. Electrical impulses enable the performance of these functions, and these impulses come from the unbalanced electron activity of free radicals. Unfortunately, excess production of free radicals interferes with the cell's ability to repair and reproduce. Excess free radicals disturb DNA and RNA synthesis, interfere with the synthesis of protein, lower energy levels, and prevent the body from building muscle mass and destroying certain cellular enzymes. Such free-radical damage begins at birth and continues until death. In early life, its effects are relatively minor because the body has extensive repair and replacement mechanisms that, in healthy young individuals, function to keep cells and organs functioning effectively. However, as individuals age, the accumulated effects of free-radical damage begin to take their toll. Free-radical disruption of cell metabolism not only ages cells but also fosters the development of chronic illness. Body organs that sustain significant free-radical damage become increasingly vulnerable to chronic disease. For example, arterial damage can lead to coronary artery disease, and excessive free-radical damage in certain brain sites can result in Alzheimer's disease or Parkinson's disease, or damaged joints can lead to the development of arthritis. When free radicals continually create mutant cells, cancer develops.

Psychological Stress and Oxidative Stress

The number of free radicals an individual produces varies from day to day, depending on his or her exposure to stressful situations. It is not just toxins in air, food, and drinking water that dramatically increase the number of free radicals produced. Just as important, intrapersonal, interpersonal, and behavioral stressors, such as excessive exercise, cigarette smoke, and alcohol and drug use, also greatly increase the number of free radicals produced. Needless to say, as biological, environmental, and psychological stressors increase, oxidative stress increases.

CULTURAL FACTORS IN CHRONIC ILLNESS

cultural factors [handwritten annotation]

Although the social dimension of the biopsychosocial model is more accurately known as the *sociocultural dimension*, it is understood as the shorthand designation for the sociocultural dimension. Needless to say, cultural issues are significant factors in health (Lewis, 2002). Cultural variables such as racial background, ethnicity, gender, sexual orientation, socioeconomic status, and ability are organizing factors of an individual's identity, lifestyle, and health status. It is axiomatic that health as well as illness behavior occurs within a cultural context. The culture of a patient can provide resources for coping with illness, as well as influence a patient's willingness to seek and accept therapeutic assistance (Canino & Guarnaccia, 1997; Leong, Wagner, & Tata, 1995). The cultural context influences how pain and discomfort are caused, experienced, and expressed, as well as the consequence of suffering (Lewis, 2002). Presumably, health-related factors vary across cultural groups. Until very recently, the idea of actively including cultural factors within the assessment and intervention process was disregarded. It was common for health professionals to fail to take a patient's cultural background into account, resulting in misattributions of behavior and lack of understanding between patient and clinician. Today, it is increasingly clear that effective, ethical, and respectful treatment is accomplished through the careful and purposeful inclusion and consideration of cultural factors and the cultural context of treatment. Those involved in providing health-focused psychotherapy and counseling must ascertain where their own cultural biases lie and look to not center treatment exclusively on themselves and their own biased cultural position (Lewis, 2002).

In short, disease does not occur within a vacuum, and chronic illness cannot be understood apart from its cultural context. It is important to note that the very concept of "illness" and the views of disease causation vary across cultures. Without an appreciation of the role of culture in the perception and manifestation of health and illness, health counselors run the risk of misinterpreting and misdiagnosing illnesses because of ethnocentric biases (Angel & Williams, 2001). Western views of disease causation are often based on naturalistic views regarding infection, stress, organic deterioration, accidents, and acts of overt aggression. In contrast, non-Western views of disease causation often have components of supernatural views regarding mystical causation (i.e., impersonal views regarding fate, ominous sensations, contagion, and so on), animistic causation due to personalized forces of soul loss and spiritual aggression, and theories of magical causation, such as witchcraft (Murdock, 1980, as cited in Marsella & Yamada, 2001). Non-Western notions of disease are seldom considered in Western professional settings, which can lead to compliance problems with those not adhering to the Western conceptualization of disease. As a rule, however, it is important to recognize that there are no set rules to determine whether responses to perception, treatment, and coping with illness will be more culturally specific than ones that appear to some as culture bound or more Western. To simply categorize responses as "Western" or "non-Western" does not allow for the understanding of other factors, including belief systems, acculturation, socioeconomic status, and other salient cultural variables (Arredondo, 1996).

Furthermore, culture exerts a profound influence on how individuals in subcultures and in the dominant culture think about disease and its treatment. Certain aspects of the dominant culture positively support and respond to individuals experiencing chronic illnesses, but others aspects of the culture make living with chronic illness very difficult. Fennell (2003) discusses six cultural factors—in the dominant culture in the United States—that are nonsupportive and even harmful to individuals with chronic illnesses. These six factors are as follows:

Intolerance of suffering: Suffering is perceived as having no value to America, and society frowns on the public expression of grief and sorrow, especially among men.

Intolerance of ambiguity: Because of their scientific bias, Americans dislike the unknowable, and much about chronic illness is unknown. This intolerance fosters feelings of powerlessness, fear that chronic disease is contagious, and the belief that people who are chronically ill are somehow responsible for their condition.

Intolerance of chronic illness: Because of their action and achievement orientation, Americans accept acute diseases because they have a distinct cause, course, treatment, and eventual cure, whereas chronic diseases do not. Furthermore, Americans have come to expect miraculous cures and technological marvels, but the nontreatability of chronic disease represents a failure of the health care system and modern medicine.

Current cultural perceptions of disease: Americans fear new diseases; for instance, recall the public hysteria surrounding AIDS in the 1980s, and those who are ill even with an "acceptable" disease are considered "outsiders" and tend to arouse suspicion.

Disease enculturation: There is a definable process in which a new disease entity is recognized and met with fear and foreboding. Later, it becomes identified and named, and after being studied and treated sufficiently, the disease entity becomes accepted as part of everyday social reality. This entire process of disease enculturation may extend over several years, and individuals who are diagnosed with the disease earlier in the process are more likely to be negatively impacted by others who contract the disease later in the enculturation process.

Influence of the media: Although the mass media can educate the public by conveying medical findings on chronic diseases, they can significantly influence and reinforce social stereotypes and cultural biases. Moreover, feature stories about a given chronic illness can result in an invasion of privacy. As Fennell (2001) described,

> Friends and co-workers have access to intimate details of your illness which you may not really want to share with them. You may not have even experienced aspects of the disease that are dramatized, but people will be convinced that you must have. (p. 25)

IMPACT OF CHRONIC ILLNESS ON THE FAMILY

Family

Chronic illness in a family member has a major impact on the family unit as a whole:

> Few health professionals or scholars challenge the proposition that illness or impairment in a family member has adverse effects on family functioning. Most agree that families of ill people generally function more poorly than families in which all the members are healthy. With the onset of an illness, the family's social life contracts and becomes primarily family centered. Within this circumscribed existence, the patient often becomes the focus of the family, with other family members forced into the background. . . . The more severe and long lasting the illness or impairment, the greater the potential for family disruption. (Turk & Kerns, 1985, p. 15)

Illness can be highly disruptive to a family's functioning, but many families do manage to cope with this stress and even become more cohesive in the process. Families that have shown a general ability to function well can continue to do so even in the wake of a serious health crisis. A family that is functioning effectively can cope with the disruption of illness and, at the same time, play an important role in supporting and assisting the affected family member. Family-focused interventions should have a dual emphasis: (a) supporting and strengthening family units as a means for enhancing the adaptation of the individual patient and (b) helping the family system as a whole maintain its functionality despite illness-related crises or challenges. Most efforts have tended to focus on the family's role in helping the affected individual achieve health stabilization or improvement.

A good example of a chronic illness that can act as a major family stressor is diabetes mellitus (DM). Following the diagnosis of DM, the patient and family often must adopt a significantly different lifestyle. In the worst of circumstances, the family must deal with an almost inevitable array of stressors, including the prospect of a shortened life span for the patient; the specter of severe complications, such as kidney failure, blindness, stroke, and amputation; apprehension over the unpredictable occurrence of insulin reactions and life-threatening crises related to ketoacidosis; and pervasive concern over the ability to handle these crises. In the best of circumstances, the family will face the daily challenge of fitting a personal and family lifestyle around monitoring and regulating the diet, exercise, and medication of their family member who has DM (Hamburg, Elliott, & Parron, 1982).

The family as a whole must make major adaptations, as would be the case with any serious illness. In the case of DM, an additional challenge is created by the urgent need for adherence to a complicated medical regimen involving a high degree of self-care. The individual affected with this disease has major health-related tasks to perform, including careful, long-term self-assessment and adherence to self-administered medical regimens that can be complex. In short, the patient with DM really needs to become his or her own physician (Hendrick, 1985). For an affected individual, treatment adherence typically involves monitoring blood sugar levels; making decisions concerning insulin injections; using oral medications; and maintaining ongoing health behaviors such as a carefully regulated diet, a weight-control regimen, and an exercise program. The family's success in adapting to the challenges of the disease may have a major effect on the individual's success in self-treatment.

The family becomes an absolutely critical ingredient in treatment if the person with DM is a child or adolescent. If the diabetic's parents are educated about the disease, offer help and support, encourage independence, stress a healthy orientation to the disease, and focus on the child rather than the disease, normal family development and interaction should follow. However, this optimum level of behavior is extremely difficult to achieve. Unfortunately, an obsessive concern with diabetic control by parents too often results either in rebelliousness or in almost overcompliance by a child. Needless to say, neither of these extremes is healthy. Conversely, denial of or lack of involvement in the treatment process by parents can be disastrous (Hendrick, 1985).

As the clinician works with the diabetic child to enhance the likelihood of adherence to treatment regimens, he or she should also work with other family members. Although knowledge of the disease is important, awareness of the challenges of self-care may have even greater significance. The more that family members understand about the nature of the self-care skills required, the more they will be able to help and support the child's efforts. Family members may also need assistance in examining their own reactions to the child's health problems so that they can balance positive concern with recognition of the child's need for control. This process is further complicated by the need to make changes in response to the child's development. As Johnson (1985) pointed out, the disease of younger children is best controlled through active parental involvement, and "giving the youngster too much responsibility too early may prove disastrous" (p. 225). In contrast, adolescents show better results if they control their own regimens. Families may need ongoing help and support if they are to adapt to constant changes in the disease itself and in the patient's psychosocial needs.

One helpful approach is to provide this assistance in the context of family support groups, which can furnish mutual nurturance along with skill development. This type of intervention may be especially useful in helping families cope with illnesses that tend to exacerbate feelings of helplessness. For example, family support groups have been used for dealing with such health problems as adult cancer (Dunkel-Schetter & Wortman, 1982; Euster, 1984), childhood cancer (Chesler & Yoak, 1984), Alzheimer's disease (Kapust & Weintraub, 1984; Kerns & Curley, 1985), spinal cord injuries (Eisenberg, 1984), and multiple sclerosis (Pavlou, 1984), all of which tend to be intensely crisis provoking.

CASE STUDY: THE IMPACT OF JUVENILE-ONSET DIABETES MELLITUS ON A FAMILY

The case that follows illustrates how chronic illness in a family member can have a major impact on the entire family. This case involves a child with a recently diagnosed chronic illness in a family that is already experiencing considerable stress.

Rachel is the 11-year-old daughter of Patricia, a widowed Caucasian woman from an upscale suburb. The mother brought Rachel and her two other daughters, Janice (age 14) and Jenny (age 7) for a consultation, complaining for 3 months that there was serious discord among her children, they were all doing poorly in school, and the oldest daughter was threatening to run away from home. In addition, the principal had notified Patricia that Rachel would be held back a year.

Some 4 months prior to this consultation, Rachel was diagnosed with juvenile-onset DM. The diagnosis was made during an emergency hospitalization after Rachel was found unconscious in her bedroom after school. The onset of diabetic symptoms was subtle and not recognized by Rachel, her family, or school personnel. At the time of this consultation, the entire family had been involved in family therapy for over 3 years, following the shooting death of Jack, Rachel's father, by her maternal grandfather. Reportedly, after learning that the grandfather had been sexually abusing Janice, Jack confronted the grandfather and told him that he was going to move his family to protect them from the grandfather. In a rage, the grandfather responded by fatally wounding the father with a rifle. Janice underwent individual therapy in addition to family therapy. Patricia indicated that many of the family sessions were directed at both sexual abuse and grieving issues. The family concluded that the treatment was only minimally effective. The purpose of the consultation was to evaluate the increasing family tension that Rachel characterized as "plain old jealousy" in Janice and Jenny. Apparently, although Rachel's DM symptoms were reasonably stabilized by insulin and diet restriction, Patricia was obsessed with finding a cure for Rachel's DM. Remarkably, whereas Rachel had come to accept her condition (her adherence to her DM self-management program was described as excellent by her physician), Patricia was in denial of the DM and was searching desperately for a miracle cure. This took the form of endless appointments to various medical specialists and alternative healers, extensive Internet searches, and phone calls to medical centers and researchers conducting trials of experimental treatments for juvenile-onset DM. This meant that she had little, if any, time to spend with her two other daughters. The way in which they behaved in the consultation suggested that Janice and Jenny were very envious of the attention Rachel received from their mother. Socially, Rachel felt somewhat awkward, given that she was much taller than her peers and because of her self-perception that somehow she was "different" as a result of her medical regimen. The regimen required three insulin injections a day, one of which was scheduled during school hours. Presumably, the endocrinologist would in time reduce this injection schedule to twice a day. For the past 3 months, there was little positive change in her health status.

The following case conceptualization is offered: The onset of Rachel's DM occurred at a time when the family was receiving family therapy as it grieved the unexpected death of the father. The extent of the family grief and the partially treated sexual abuse of the oldest daughter appeared to have overly stressed this close-knit family sufficiently enough to express the DM in Rachel, the most medically vulnerable family member. The DM serves to restore some measure of family cohesion by mobilizing family members to "control and cure" the identified patient's symptoms, given that a basic theme of the family's narrative is that "caring means controlling." Unfortunately, the mother's seeming overconcern with finding a miracle cure appears to be exacerbating family turmoil. The impact of Rachel's DM on her family is assessed as moderate–severe, and the focal conflict was sibling jealousy over the attention that the mother was giving to Rachel at the expense of the other two daughters. The resulting decline in academic performance of all the children, increasing conflict, and decreasing family cohesion are notable. Without the likely buffering effect of their ongoing family therapy, the situation would most likely be considerably worse. Nevertheless, until the mother is able to more equitably attend to the needs of the oldest and youngest daughters, jealousy and discord will continue.

CONCLUDING NOTE

As psychology—particularly the clinically oriented areas, including psychotherapy—revises itself as a primary health care specialty, the biopsychosocial perspective will eventually replace the psychosocial perspective. This chapter has emphasized the need for, and clinical value and use of, the biopsychosocial model in understanding and treating chronic illness. The complex and reciprocal relationship among biological, personality, and psychosocial factors and processes has been emphasized, articulated, and explained with a serious degenerative chronic disease, rheumatoid arthritis. Biopsychosocial features of other common chronic diseases are described in chapter 3. Because personality is another key factor in the biopsychosocial model presented in this chapter, its impact on the chronic illness process is detailed in chapter 4.

3

BIOPSYCHOSOCIAL ASPECTS OF SOME COMMON CHRONIC ILLNESSES

Although there are over <u>100 chronic diseases</u>, there are a few that are quite common among adults in the United States. These include arthritis, asthma, cancer, chronic fatigue syndrome (CFS), chronic sinusitis, diabetes mellitus (DM), epilepsy, hypertension, irritable bowel syndrome (IBS), and systemic lupus erythematosus (SLE). Fortunately, <u>the progression</u> of each of these diseases can be greatly attenuated, particularly in the early stages, with effective health counseling and psychotherapy strategies. Psychotherapists who are working or are planning to work with individuals who are chronically ill need a basic understanding of both the disease states and the experience of the particular illnesses of these individuals. This chapter provides a focused description of both the disease process and the illness experience for these 10 common chronic conditions.

Each of these diseases is discussed in terms of its clinical description, symptoms, prevalence, course of progression, medical treatment, and patient education and self-management. Much of the information on these disease conditions is from the National Center for Chronic Disease Prevention and Health Promotion's (2000) recent publication *Chronic Diseases and Their Risk Factors: The Nation's Leading Causes of Death, 1999*).[1]

---

[1]Readers seeking additional information on these and other chronic diseases may find two of the Merck manuals readily available in most bookstores and libraries and very readable. The first is *The Merck Manual of Diagnosis and Therapy* (17th ed.; Beers & Berkow, 1999), which has been a standard medical reference source for allied health professionals for over 100 years. The second is *The Merck Manual of Medical Information* (2nd ed.; Beers, 2003), which is billed as the world's most widely used medical reference and is written in everyday language.

DESCRIPTIONS OF 10 COMMON CHRONIC DISEASES

Arthritis

Arthritis is a chronic condition of the joints. There are two types: osteoarthritis and rheumatoid arthritis. This section emphasizes osteoarthritis, which is by far the more prevalent condition. Osteoarthritis affects approximately 65% of older adults, whereas rheumatoid arthritis affects only about 5% of the total population. Osteoarthritis alters the hyaline cartilage and causes loss of the articular cartilage of the joint, as well as irregular growth to the connecting bone structures. This disease begins asymptomatically before age 40, and afterwards nearly everyone who has it experiences some pathological changes in their weight-bearing joints. Although men and women are equally affected by it, the onset is sooner in men. Pain is the earliest reported symptom and is increased by exercise and relieved by rest. Morning stiffness lasts 10 to 30 minutes and lessens with movement. As the disease progresses, joint motion decreases, and tenderness and grating sounds—called *crepitus*—appear. As articular cartilage is lost in the joint, ligaments become lax. Ligaments that effectively supported the joint before the disease progressed now become lax or loosened, resulting in the joint becoming less stable and increasing the risk of complications, such as fractures, if the individual falls. Pain and tenderness are experienced, arising from the changes in the ligaments and tendons.

Osteoarthritis, rheumatoid arthritis, and other joint conditions affect nearly 43 million Americans, which is about 1 of every 6 individuals. As the nation's population ages, arthritis is expected to affect 60 million people by 2020. Osteoarthritis has the distinction of being the largest single cause of disability in the United States. It is characterized by its uncertain prognosis, its uncertain course, and its significant psychosocial impact. It is estimated to cost almost $65 billion annually in medical care and lost productivity. Although prevailing myths have portrayed arthritis as an inevitable part of aging that can only be endured, effective interventions are available to prevent or reduce arthritis-related pain and disability.

Medical treatment includes medications to reduce inflammation, pain, and swelling, as well as physical therapy and exercise. Rehabilitation techniques are also used, for the purpose of preventing dysfunction and decreasing the severity or duration of disability. It is interesting to note that psychological factors are more strongly associated with disability than is the disease process itself.

Self-management appears to be an important part of the treatment regimen. Usually, this involves a patient education component in which information about the disease and its manifestation and progressive course is provided. This can be accomplished in face-to-face contact, with phone contact, or by computer programs or written materials. In addition, strategies such as exercise, relaxation training, skill training in cognitive pain management, problem solving, and social skills can be incorporated. These strategies can be learned over a period of weeks in a classroom, a small group, or an individual context. Typically, cognitive strategies such as cognitive pain management focus on reframing the individual's way of thinking about the disease and on modulating the chronic pain component. Because of the significant psychological component, counseling and referral for psychotherapy are common intervention choices today.

Asthma

Asthma is a chronic respiratory disease. It is characterized by a reversible airway obstruction and airway responsiveness to a variety of irritants. It is usually accompanied by tissue inflammation, mucus congestion, and constriction of the smooth muscles in the airways. Whether caused by airway edema, acute bronchoconstriction, chronic mucus plugs, or changes in the lung itself, airflow obstruction and airflow hyperresponsiveness are signature features of this disease. Airway obstruction is due to a combination of factors, including spasm of airway smooth muscles, edema of airway mucosa, increased mucus secretion, or infiltration of the airway walls. The end result is an "asthma attack." Although there is great variability in symptomatology, an asthma attack begins with spasms of wheezing, coughing, and shortness of breath. Tightness or pressure in the chest and wheezing may also be present.

The prevalence of asthma in the United States is about 5% among adults and 7% among children, although the incidence appears to be increasing. Morbidity and mortality increase disproportionately among the indigent in inner-city areas. Approximately 25% of those with asthma experience severe symptoms. Of this, the greater majority are women, ethnic minorities, those with little education, smokers, and those receiving care from nonspecialists. In comparison to those with mild to moderate asthma, those with severe symptoms also tend to have less of an understanding of the asthma, its clinical manifestations, and the means to control asthma attacks. Asthma is the leading cause of hospitalization among children and is responsible for more absenteeism from school than any other chronic illness.

Just as symptoms are varied, the experience of this disease state varies widely. Most commonly—in at least 50% of cases—people with asthma experience a reaction within seconds after exposure to a trigger, and this reaction continues for approximately 1 hour. There is also a delayed reaction that begins 4 to 8 hours after exposure, which lasts for hours or even days.

Chronic inflammation causes the airways of these individuals to become hyperresponsive to allergens, physical exertion, cigarette smoke, molds, and even breathing cold air. Psychological factors, including crying, screaming, failed expectations, or relational stress, may trigger symptoms.

The course of this disease is highly variable, depending on the individual's unique symptoms, triggers or precipitants of symptoms, health status, and capacity for self-management of the condition. Thus, it should not be too surprising that nearly 75% of emergency room admissions for asthma are avoidable. Furthermore, approximately 40% of people with asthma do not use appropriate symptom management strategies when their symptoms worsen. Upwards of 60% of people with asthma are poor at judging the extent of *dyspnea*, which is the subjective difficulty or distress in breathing.

Effective medical treatment usually involves a management protocol. It consists of assessing the severity of the illness, controlling environmental factors to avoid or minimize triggering symptoms or exacerbations, using medication to manage exacerbations and to reverse and prevent airway inflammation, using patient education and self-management methods, and monitoring the course of therapy. The goal of medical treatment is to prevent chronic symptoms, maintain pulmonary or lung function as near to normal as possible, prevent exacerbations, minimize the need for emergency room visits and hospitalization, and avoid the adverse effects of treatment. Recovery from this condition is typically defined as movement into the normal range of pulmonary function. Needless to say, even small improvements can be clinically significant. The focus of traditional medical treatment is entirely on management rather than on cure.

Self-management is a key component in effective asthma management. It involves at least two goals. The first goal is to assist these individuals to self-manage their asthma at home and to work through treatment adjustments in response to changes in their symptoms. Patient education is a necessary prerequisite for effective self-management. It includes basic facts about asthma, the role of quick-response and long-term control medications, the correct use of metered-dose inhalers, strategies for decreasing environmental exposure, a reduction plan for acute episodes, and the involvement of family and significant others in the treatment process. Equally important is the second goal, which is the development of the patient's skills, judgment, and confidence necessary for engaging in self-management activities and for collaborating with health care providers.

Cancer

Cancer, or *malignancy*, refers to any of the more than 100 diseases characterized by excessive, uncontrolled growth of abnormal cells. Cancer invades and destroys other adjacent tissues and metastasizes, that is, spreads to other regions of the body. Cancer can develop in any tissue of any organ at any age.

Each year, more than 1.2 million Americans are diagnosed with cancer. It is the second-leading cause of death among Americans, causing an estimated 550,000 U.S. deaths in 2000. It is estimated that 8.4 million Americans alive today have a history of cancer, and about 1,200 Americans die from cancer each day. Cancer costs this nation an estimated $107 billion annually in health care expenditures and lost productivity. For reasons not well understood, cancer rates vary by gender, race, and geographic region. For instance, more males have cancer than females, and African Americans are more likely to develop cancer than persons of any other racial and ethnic group in the United States. Cancer rates also vary globally—residents of the United States, for example, are nearly 3 times as likely to develop cancer as are residents of Egypt.

Researchers from Columbia University School of Public Health reported that 95% of cancer is caused by diet and environment (Perera, 1997). As with other chronic diseases in which individuals' lifestyle choices interact with their genes, cancer is in large part a controllable disease. In fact, most cancers are potentially curable if detected at an early stage. By performing self-examinations, individuals can help recognize early signs of some cancers. Diagnostic testing and therapy are essential for optimal results. When cure or reasonable management is likely, the physicians should discuss all therapeutic options. Reducing the incidence of cancer requires that the behavioral and environmental factors that increase cancer risk be addressed and that screening and health counseling services be made available and accessible in its early, most treatable stages.

Individuals with cancers that are unlikely to be cured need to be informed about what treatments are likely to accomplish and which side effects can be expected. Intensive care may be needed for treatment-related complications. Psychological support helps individuals tolerate, as well as profit from, cancer treatment, particularly when it involves severe side effects.

More than 100 types of cancer have been identified according to the site at which the cancer originates, the type of tissue, and the type of cell. Thus, *lung cancer* describes any cancer that originated in the lung. If the cancer spreads to a new organ, such as the liver, the tumor is called *metastatic lung cancer*, not *liver cancer*.

Each body organ is composed of different types of tissue, and most cancers arise in one of three main types of tissue—epithelial, connective, or blood forming. *Carcinomas* are cancers that occur in epithelial tissues—the skin and inner membrane surfaces, such as those of the lungs, stomach, intestines, and blood vessels. Carcinomas account for approximately 90% of human cancers. *Sarcomas*, which account for less than 2% of all cancers, originate in connective tissues, that is, muscle, bone, cartilage, and fat that connect body parts. *Leukemia* develops in blood cells, and lymphomas originate in the lymphatic system. Combined, these cancers account for the remaining 8%.

Cancers are further identified according to the type of cell affected. Cancers that originate from *squamous cells*, that is, flat, scalelike cells found in epithelial tissue, are called *squamous cell carcinomas*. *Adenomatous cells* are glandular or ductal cells, and carcinomas that originate in these cells are called *adenocarcinomas*. Furthermore, sarcomas that develop in fat cells are called *liposarcomas*, and those that develop in bone cells are called *osteosarcomas*.

Typical early symptoms of cancer include fatigue, weight loss, fevers, night sweats, a cough, bloody stools or a change in bowel habits, and persistent pain. Necessary to early diagnosis of cancer is a complete history and physical examination. The purpose of cancer screening and early diagnosis is to decrease cancer mortality, to allow the use of less radical therapies, and to reduce the financial cost. Common screening procedures include the Pap smear for cervical cancer, breast examination and mammography for breast cancer, and the PSA blood test and digital rectal exam for prostate cancer.

Successful treatment of cancer requires an elimination of all cancer cells, whether at the primary site, in adjacent areas, or as metastases to other regions of the body. The major medical modalities of treatment are surgery, radiation, and chemotherapy. Other methods include endocrine therapy for selected cancers such as breast, prostate, or liver cancer; immunotherapies; and multimodal therapy, which combine the assets of two or more of these modalities.

Researchers estimate that more than 60% of cancer deaths in the United States are preventable through lifestyle changes. Although there is no certain way to avoid all cancers, reducing individual risk factors significantly decreases the likelihood of contracting many forms of this devastating disease. The American Cancer Society estimates that smoking causes nearly 30% of all cancer deaths in the United States, that is, approximately 166,000 cancer deaths each year. In short, all cancer deaths caused by cigarette smoking could be prevented completely by not smoking and not using smokeless tobacco. For those who already smoke, quitting will reduce the risk of developing cancer. After about 10 years of not smoking, a former smoker's risk lowers to that of a nonsmoker.

Next to quitting smoking, eating a healthy diet is the best way to lower the risk of cancer. Specific foods have been shown to protect against cancer, such as broccoli, cauliflower, cabbage, tomatoes, and soy products, as well as foods high in vitamins A, C, and E. In addition, green teas contain antioxidants that protect the body from carcinogens. Antioxidants work by blocking the action of free radicals. Other chemicals in fruits and vegetables are thought to block the cell-growth-promoting effects of steroid hormones, protecting against cancers of the prostate and breast.

Diets that include limited amounts of red meat appear to lower the risk of cancer. Other foods to avoid or consume in moderation include sugar, saturated animal fat, and salt. Dietary fats and oils should come from vegetables, such as olives or corn, rather than from animal sources. Carbohydrates should come from whole grains, such as brown rice and whole wheat bread, rather than from processed foods, such as white rice and white bread. The risk of cancer of the esophagus increases with heavy alcohol consumption, and research suggests that the use of alcohol increases the risk of breast cancer as well.

Low levels of physical activity have been implicated in colon cancer. Moderate activity for 30 minutes a day enhances the immune system, shortens the time food takes to move through the intestines, and alters body composition and hormone levels. Physical activity also helps avoid obesity, which is associated with an increased risk for cancers of the colon and rectum, prostate, breast, endometrium, and kidney. Maintaining a healthy weight through regular physical activity and a healthy diet, individuals can substantially lower their risk for these cancers. Furthermore, protecting the skin from the sun's rays could prevent about 80% of all skin cancers. Practicing safe sex can also reduce cancer risk. The human papilloma virus (HPV), linked to cervical cancer, is the most common cancer-causing virus in the United States. Limiting the number of sexual partners, using condoms, or practicing sexual abstinence reduces the risk of infection with HPV. Infection with the human immunodeficiency virus (HIV), also sexually transmitted, greatly increases an individual's risk for cancers of the immune and lymphatic system, such as Kaposi's sarcoma. Infection with the Hepatitis B virus is the predominant cause of liver cancer in the United States.

Chronic Fatigue Syndrome

CFS is a clinically defined condition characterized by severe disabling fatigue and a combination of symptoms that prominently features self-reported impairments in concentration and short-term memory, sleep disturbances, and musculoskeletal pain. CFS is a relatively recently defined condition and remains somewhat of a controversial medical condition. Because its diagnosis is made only after alternate medical and psychiatric causes of chronic fatiguing illness have been ruled out, it is referred to as a "diagnosis by exclusion." Even though there are no *pathognomonic*—that is, characteristic and definitive—signs of this disorder, and no diagnostic tests are currently available, the following definition was developed by a national task force and published in the prestigious *Annals of Internal Medicine* and is accepted by many in the medical community: CFS is defined by the presence of (a) clinically evaluated, unexplained persistent or relapsing chronic fatigue that is of new or definite onset (i.e., has not been lifelong); is not the result of ongoing exertion; is not substantially alleviated by rest; and results in substantial reduction in previous levels of occupational, educational, social, or personal activities; and (b) the concurrent occurrence of four or more of the following symptoms, all of which must have persisted or recurred during 6 or more consecutive months of illness and must not have predated the fatigue: self-reported impairment in short-term memory or concentration severe enough to cause a substantial reduction in previous levels of occupational, educational, social, or personal activities; sore throat; tender cervical or auxiliary lymph nodes; muscle pain; multijoint pain without joint swelling or redness; headaches of a new type, pattern, or severity; nonrefreshing sleep; and postexertional malaise lasting more than 24 hours (Fukuda et al., 1994). At this point, the matter of specifying risk factors for CFS is uncertain. Although CFS was originally thought to be triggered by the Epstein–Barr virus, which causes mononucleosis, or other viruses such as herpes and polio, CFS has been shown to be noncontiguous. There is growing speculation that the actual cause is a combination of a weakened immune system and the presence of a virus and one or more of the following risk factors: chronic candidiasis; a history of recurrent use of antibiotics or *nonsteroidal anti-inflammatory drugs* (NSAIDs), that is, the class of drugs such as Tylenol, Motrin, and Celebrex; chronic infections, such as sinusitis or prostatitis; chemical exposure or sensitivity to cigarette smoke, perfume or paint fumes, or other chemicals; leaky gut syndrome; a diet high in sugar and caffeine; and so on.

Because there is no specific laboratory test or clinical sign for CFS, accurate prevalence data are not available. However, the Centers for Disease Control and Prevention (CDC) estimates that as many as 500,000 people in the United States have CFS or a CFS-like condition. It has also been observed that CFS is diagnosed 2 to 4 times more often in women than in men.

For many, CFS begins either after a minor illness such as a cold or the flu or during a period of high stress. Unlike flu symptoms, which usually go away in a few days or weeks, CFS symptoms continue on and off for more than 6 months. Reported symptoms include headache, tender lymph nodes, fatigue and weakness, muscle and joint aches, and inability to concentrate. The course of CFS varies from person to person. For most, CFS symptoms reach a certain level and become stable early in the course of illness and thereafter come and go. Some individuals get better completely, but it is not clear how frequently this happens. Emotional support and counseling can help the individual and significant others cope with the uncertain outlook and the waxing and waning of symptoms and the energy level of this illness.

Medical treatment may include a trial of an antiviral drug such as Zovirax. Antidepressants sometimes help to improve sleep and relieve mild, general pain. Some individuals benefit from other drugs for acute anxiety or for dizziness and extreme tenderness in the skin.

Although self-management protocols are still being developed, several health behaviors appear to be useful in symptom reduction and even resolution of the condition. These include a balanced diet; adequate rest; regular exercise that does not cause more fatigue; limiting stress; pacing oneself physically, emotionally, and intellectually; and emotional and spiritual health recommendations. The use of psychosocial interventions is also recommended (Friedberg & Jason, 1998).

A balanced, whole-foods diet—that is, one emphasizing quality proteins and complex carbohydrates such as organic vegetables, whole grains, beans, fish, eggs, and poultry—is recommended. Sugar, caffeine, dairy products, alcohol, aspartame, and refined carbohydrates, such as white flour and rice, are to be avoided. Walking and mild aerobic exercise, along with mild stretching, is the preferred exercise regimen. Because psychological factors, particularly depression, can be prominent, a number of mental and emotional health techniques may be indicated, including stress reduction methods such as controlled breathing and biofeedback (Baum & Andersen, 2001). Other techniques include massage and bodywork therapies, journaling, planned retreats and vacations, and creative activities such as art and music. Because CFS involves a depletion of life-force energy, it can be thought of as a spiritual condition. Some spiritual disciplines or techniques, such as prayer, meditation, gratitude and acceptance, and forgiveness, might serve to strengthen the individual's immune system.

Chronic Sinusitis

Sinusitis is an infection or inflammation of the lining of one or more of the eight sinus cavities in the facial bones around the nose. It usually begins as a cold and is accompanied by most or all of the primary symptoms of head congestion; headache or pressurelike pain on the forehead, temples, cheeks, or nose, or around or behind the eyes; facial pain; difficulty breathing through the nose; a thick yellow or greenish discharge that drains into the nose or down the back of the throat; and fatigue. Most cases of sinusitis are acute sinusitis, which lasts less than 4 weeks. However, signs and symptoms of sinusitis lasting more than 12 weeks is indicative of chronic sinusitis. *Recurrent sinusitis* refers to several acute attacks within a year. Chronic sinusitis can also be diagnosed if the individual has one of the major signs or symptoms and at least two of the following minor signs or symptoms: aching in the upper jaw and teeth, bad breath, ear pain, or a cough. The definitive medical diagnosis of sinusitis is determined with a magnetic resonance imaging (MRI) or computed tomography (CT) scan of the sinuses.

Chronic sinusitis is one of the most common chronic diseases in the United States, affecting an estimated 33 million individuals a year, of which 29.2 million are adults. In 2002, this meant that 14.2% were diagnosed with sinusitis. The condition accounted for 12.3 million visits to office-based physicians in 2001 and 1.1 million hospital outpatient visits in 2002.

The causes of chronic sinusitis are only recently being clarified. In nearly all cases, the nasal and sinus mucosa become so inflamed that sinuses cannot drain properly, and microorganisms such as viruses, bacteria, or fungi multiply and cause infection. Infection causes swelling, which further reduces sinus drainage. For years, it was believed that bacteria were the primary causative factor. The publication of a widely publicized research report in 1999

(Ponika, Sherris, & Kern, 1999) changed that belief. The report concluded that the cause of most cases of chronic sinusitis was an immune system response to fungus rather than bacteria. Researchers at the Mayo Clinic concluded this after studying 210 patients with chronic sinusitis and discovering 40 different fungi, including candida, in the mucus of 96% of them (Ponika et al., 1999). Thus, the cause of much, if not most, chronic sinusitis is inflamed mucosa and an overly reactive immune response to fungi in the sinus cavities.

Other factors that promote sinus blockage are allergic disease or sensitivity to airborne allergens, such as dust, mold, and pollen. Those prone to chronic sinusitis can be sensitive to damp weather, especially in northern temperate climates, or to pollutants in the air and in buildings. Furthermore, those with an immune deficiency disease or an abnormality in the way mucus moves through and from their respiratory system—for instance, immune deficiency, HIV infection, and cystic fibrosis—can develop chronic sinusitis. Those with severe asthma, nasal polyps (i.e., small growths in the nose), or a severe asthmatic response to aspirin and aspirin-like medicines such as ibuprofen can develop chronic sinusitis. Finally, trauma such as a fractured facial bone that obstructs one or more sinus cavities can confound this medical condition.

Chronic sinusitis can be difficult to diagnose because the symptoms may be very similar to colds or allergies. The experience of most individuals is that they have had chronic sinusitis for several years before it is properly diagnosed. Typically, individuals have come to believe their symptoms were due to a cold or allergy, or they had several episodes of acute sinusitis that were not properly treated and, as a result, developed chronic sinusitis. Chronic sinusitis can increase the frequency and severity of asthmatic flare-ups in those with asthma and in those who have asthma-like reactions to aspirin and related medications such as ibuprofen.

Physicians have found that successful treatment of chronic sinusitis has been elusive, because symptoms often persist after long periods of antibiotic treatment, that is, a minimum of 3 weeks and up to 12 weeks. Previously, it was assumed that treating chronic sinusitis should be similar to treating acute sinusitis, for which antibiotics and decongestants are used. Unfortunately, fungi rather than bacteria are causative factors in chronic sinusitis in most cases. Newer protocols substituted antifungal medications such as Nizoral or Diflucan for antibiotics. Commonly prescribed decongestants include Seldane and Claritin. Because corticosteroids can reduce massive inflammation, nasal corticosteroid sprays or oral corticosteroids are prescribed to shrink the inflamed sinus membranes. These corticasteroids include Beconase, Nasacort, and Vancenase. When antibiotics and decongestants failed to improve the situation, surgery was often recommended. Typically, surgery is used to enlarge a narrow sinus passage or to remove a bone or polyp that is blocking a sinus passage from draining. The most common surgery done today is functional endoscopic sinus surgery, in which the natural openings from the sinuses are enlarged to allow drainage.

Although self-management protocols for chronic sinusitis are limited at the present time, there is one that bears mention. Called *sinus survival*, this protocol that involves both conventional and integrative medicine interventions shows promise. Early research suggests its efficacy (Ivker, 2000). The goals of the protocol are to heal nasal and sinus mucosa, to strengthen the immune system, and to reduce the level of fungal organisms in the respiratory system. The protocol involves prevention measures, nutritional supplements, and specific medications—for instance, antifungal medications and so on.

Individuals are helped to assess and reduce their risk of chronic sinusitis by carefully treating allergies and colds. Often that means avoiding cigarette, cigar, and pipe smoke and other air pollutants that can cause sinus membranes to swell. Inhaling steam from a vaporizer, saline nasal spray, and nasal irrigation can soothe inflamed sinus cavities, as can increasing water intake and the use of a humidifier if room air is heated by a dry forced-air system. Air-conditioning air filters are helpful in removing allergens from the air. Because alcohol causes nasal and sinus membranes to swell, reducing alcohol consumption is helpful. A number of psychosocial strategies are included in this protocol. These include the following: stress management; positive affirmations; dealing with unexpressed emotions, particularly anger; and centering exercises, such as controlled breathing, meditation, and enhancing close, intimate relationships (Ivkar, 2000).

Diabetes Mellitus

DM, commonly referred to as *diabetes*, is a syndrome characterized by *hyperglycemia*, that is, high levels of glucose or sugar in the blood, resulting in varying degrees of impairment in insulin secretion or insulin action or both. Individuals with Type 1 diabetes—also known as *insulin-dependent diabetes* or *juvenile-onset diabetes*—can develop diabetic ketoacidosis, that is, an accumulation of ketones in the blood, which can result in diabetic coma and death if not aggressively treated. Individuals with Type 2 diabetes—also known as *noninsulin-dependent diabetes*—may develop a nonketotic type of coma. In either type, severe complications can develop, including coronary artery disease, blindness, kidney failure, and peripheral neuropathy. Early presentation of this disease is variable, ranging from weight loss (Type 1) to weight gain (Type 2), and is often diagnosed in asymptomatic individuals during a routine medical exam by screening blood and urine tests.

An estimated 16 million Americans have diabetes, of which two thirds have been diagnosed. That means that approximately one third of them do not know they have a serious, chronic disease. Approximately 90% have Type 2 diabetes, which has been associated with obesity in adults and, more recently, even with obesity in adolescents and children. About 1,700 new cases are diagnosed every day in the United States. Diabetes is the seventh-leading cause of death among Americans. It is the leading cause of new cases of blindness, kidney failure, and lower extremity amputations. It also greatly increases a person's risk for heart attack or stroke. Diabetes accounts for more than $98 billion in direct and indirect medical costs and lost productivity each year. It could be prevented with early detection, improved delivery of care, and psychosocial interventions.

Medical treatment of Type 1 diabetes includes insulin, diet, and patient education. Because hyperglycemia is responsible for most of the long-term complications of diabetes and because insulin can effectively control blood glucose levels, insulin has become the primary medical treatment. Diet is also useful in maintaining acceptable glucose levels. Patient education, together with diet and exercise, is essential in maintaining effective glucose control. Educational efforts are essential in engaging the patient with diabetes in a self-management program, which traditionally consists of glucose monitoring and food intake monitoring. The medical treatment of Type 2 diabetes begins with patient education, diet, exercise, and self-management. Diet plans generally involve low-fat diets that are tailored to the individual's lifestyle, ethnicity, and culture. The goal is to achieve weight reduction in overweight individuals with Type 2 diabetes. Unfortunately, only about 10% of those with Type 2 have been able to control their diabetes with diet and exercise alone. For most of the rest, having diabetes means that insulin injections are needed to achieve acceptable blood sugar control.

Self-management programs for diabetes are the most developed of any other type of self-management program for chronic disease (Redman, 2004). There is also considerable research on factors that facilitate and hinder success in diabetic self-management efforts. For instance, eating disorders are relatively common in female adolescents attempting to adjust insulin levels to control their weight. Similarly, anxiety disorders are reported to be more prevalent in people with diabetes who have poor insulin control. In addition, clinical depression is noted in 15% to 20% of those with diabetes and also interferes with adequate self-management of their diabetes (Redman, 2004). Adolescents appear to lack the cognitive ability to manipulate the various aspects of a diabetes self-management program (Schilling, Grey, & Knafl, 2002), and family dynamics can significantly impact control of their blood sugar. When there is greater cohesion and less conflict, children and adolescents experience fewer episodes of ketoacidosis and severe hypoglycemia (Gonder-Frederick, Cox, & Ritterband, 2002).

Research on personal health beliefs and self-efficacy is predictive of success or failure in self-management efforts (Redman, 2004). Studies have shown that the personal representations of diabetes by those with the illness are strongly associated with their self-management efforts. Specifically, their beliefs concerning the seriousness of their illness and the effectiveness of their treatment are most predictive of their blood sugar control and diet control (Redman, 2004). A major challenge in both traditional medical treatment regimens and self-management efforts is the matter of food intake, that is, the choice of eating when and whatever the individual wants to eat or not eat can influence an individual's sense of self-efficacy.

Epilepsy

Epilepsy is a brain disorder in which clusters of nerve cells, or neurons, in the brain fire abnormally. In epilepsy, the normal pattern of neuronal activity becomes disturbed, causing strange sensations, emotions, and behavior, or sometimes convulsions, muscle spasms, and loss of consciousness. During a seizure, neurons may fire as many as 500 times a second, much faster than the normal rate of about 80 times a second. In some people, this happens only occasionally; in others, it may happen up to hundreds of times a day. More than 2 million people in the United States, which is about 1% of the population, have experienced an unprovoked seizure or have been diagnosed with epilepsy. For about 80% of those diagnosed with epilepsy, seizures can be controlled with medication or surgery. However, about 20% of people with epilepsy will continue to experience seizures, that is, intractable epilepsy, even with the best available treatment. Experiencing a seizure does not necessarily mean that a person has epilepsy, because two or more witnessed seizures are required for the diagnosis of epilepsy.

Epilepsy is not contagious, nor is it caused by mental illness or mental retardation. Seizures sometimes do cause brain damage, particularly if they are severe, but most seizures do not seem to have a detrimental effect on the brain. Although epilepsy cannot currently be cured, for some people it does eventually go away. The odds of becoming seizure free are not as good for adults or for children with severe epilepsy syndromes, but it is nonetheless possible that seizures may decrease or even stop over time. This is more likely if the epilepsy has been well controlled by medication or if the person has epilepsy surgery.

Epilepsy is a disorder with many possible causes. Anything that disturbs the normal pattern of neuron activity—from illness to brain damage to abnormal brain development—can lead to seizures. It may develop because of an abnormality in brain wiring, an imbalance of neurotransmitters, or some combination of these factors. Researchers believe that some people with epilepsy have an abnormally high level of excitatory neurotransmitters that increase neuronal activity, although others have an abnormally low level of inhibitory neurotransmitters that decrease neuronal activity in the brain. In some cases, the brain's attempts to repair itself after a head injury, stroke, or other problem may inadvertently generate abnormal nerve connections that lead to epilepsy. Abnormalities in brain wiring that occur during brain development also may disturb neuronal activity and lead to epilepsy. About half of all seizures have no known cause. However, in other cases, the seizures are clearly linked to infection, poisoning, head injury, or other identifiable problems.

Although more than 30 different types of seizures have been identified, seizures are divided into two major categories—focal seizures and generalized seizures. Focal seizures, also called partial seizures, occur in just one part of the brain. About 60% of people with epilepsy have focal seizures. These seizures are frequently described by the area of the brain in which they originate. The symptoms of focal seizures can easily be confused with those of other disorders. For instance, the dreamlike perceptions associated with a complex focal seizure may be misdiagnosed as migraine headaches, which also may cause a dreamlike state. The strange behavior and sensations caused by focal seizures also can be mistaken for symptoms of narcolepsy, fainting, or even mental illness. It may require extensive testing and careful monitoring by a specialist to differentiate between epilepsy and other disorders.

Generalized seizures are a result of abnormal neuronal activity on both sides of the brain. They may cause loss of consciousness, falls, or massive muscle spasms. There are many kinds of generalized seizures. In absence seizures, also called *petit mal seizures*, the individual may appear to be staring into space or to have jerking or twitching muscles. *Tonic seizures* cause stiffening of muscles of the body, generally those in the back, legs, and arms. Chronic seizures cause repeated jerking movements of muscles on both sides of the body. *Myoclonic seizures* cause jerks or twitches of the upper body, arms, or legs. *Atonic seizures* cause a loss of normal muscle tone. The affected person will fall down or may drop his or her head involuntarily. *Tonic-clonic seizures* cause a mixture of symptoms, including stiffening of the body and repeated jerks of the arms or legs as well as loss of consciousness. Tonic-clonic seizures are sometimes referred to by an older term: *grand mal seizures*.

Not all seizures can be easily defined as either focal or generalized. Some people have seizures that begin as focal seizures but then spread to the entire brain. Others may have focal or generalized seizures but with no clear pattern. Three other types commonly noted in behavioral health settings are *temporal lobe epilepsy (TLE)*, *febrile seizures*, and *psychogenic seizures*. Psychogenic seizures are covered in detail at the end of this section.

TLE is the most common epilepsy syndrome with focal seizures. These seizures are often associated with auras and typically begin in childhood. Research has shown that repeated temporal lobe seizures can cause the hippocampus, important for memory and learning, to shrink over time. Although it may take years of temporal lobe seizures for measurable hippocampal damage to occur, this finding underlines the need to treat TLE early and as effectively as possible.

It is not uncommon in a patient's medical history to find mention of *febrile seizures*, which refer to seizures in childhood occurring during the course of an acute illness with a high fever. However, most children who have a febrile seizure do not develop epilepsy; the risk of subsequent nonfebrile seizures is only 2% to 3%, unless one of these factors is present.

A number of different tests are used to diagnose this chronic disease. These include electroencephalogram (EEG) monitoring, brain scans, and various blood tests, as well as developmental, neurological, and behavioral tests. Accurate diagnosis of the type of epilepsy a person has is crucial for finding an effective treatment. There are many different ways to treat epilepsy. Currently available treatments can control seizures at least some of the time in about 80% of people with epilepsy. However, another 20%—about 600,000 people with epilepsy in the United States—have intractable seizures, and another 400,000 feel they get inadequate relief from available treatments. These statistics make it clear that improved treatments are desperately needed.

The most common approach to treating epilepsy is to prescribe antiepileptic drugs. More than 20 different antiepileptic drugs are used; the choice of drug used depends on factors such as the type and frequency of seizures, the person's lifestyle and age, and so on. Most seizures can be controlled with one drug at the optimal dosage; however, a combination of drugs is used when monotherapy fails to effectively control a patient's seizures. When seizures cannot be adequately controlled by medications, surgery may be recommended. Surgery is used to remove the *seizure focus*, that is, the small area of the brain where seizures originate, or to treat underlying conditions, that is, cases in which seizures are caused by a brain tumor, hydrocephalus, or other condition. Once the underlying condition is successfully treated, seizures may remit, that is, disappear. When seizures originate in a part of the brain that cannot be removed, surgeons may implant a vagus nerve stimulator or use magnetic cranial stimulation, in which a strong magnet is held outside the head to influence brain activity in hopes of reducing seizure activity.

Diet modification may be helpful in reducing seizure activity. Maintaining a diet rich in fats and low in carbohydrates, called the *ketogenic diet*, causes the body to break down fats instead of carbohydrates, resulting in a condition called *ketosis*, which has been associated with reduced seizure activity. The efficacy of this treatment option appears to be mixed.

Individuals with epilepsy, especially children, can develop behavioral and emotional problems. Those with epilepsy have an increased risk of poor self-esteem, depression, and suicide. Individual therapy and family counseling can be valuable in increasing coping capacity and resolving conflicts. Another important component of self-management of this chronic illness is epilepsy support groups, which provide individuals and family members a venue in which to process their experiences, fears, and frustrations and to learn new coping skills.

Psychogenic Seizures

Psychogenic seizures, also called *pseudoseizures*, are not usually classified as epilepsy, although they can occur in individuals who have, or in those who do not have, epilepsy. Persons of all ages may experience psychogenic seizures, and they occur 3 times more frequently in females than in males. They may arise from various psychological factors, such as suggestion or the desire to be excused from work, to collect financial compensation, or to escape an intolerable social situation and are triggered by a conscious or unconscious desire for increased care and attention, anxiety, or pain. It is notable that they seldom occur in the absence of others.

Psychogenic seizures start with rapid breathing that leads to a buildup of carbon dioxide and thus can cause symptoms remarkably similar to *epileptic seizures*, that is, prickling in the face, hands, and feet; stiffening; trembling; writhing and thrashing movements; quivering; screaming or talking sounds; and falling to the floor. Psychogenic attacks differ from epileptic seizures in that out-of-phase movements of the upper and lower extremities, pelvic thrusting, and side-to-side head movements are evident. However, they vary from one occurrence to another and are not readily stereotyped. Indicators like papillary dilation, depressed corneal reflexes, and the presence of the Babinski reflex, autonomic cardiorespiratory changes, and tongue biting and urinary or fecal incontinence are more likely seen in epilepsy but are seldom manifested in psychogenic seizures. These attacks may last a few minutes or hours, and they may end as abruptly as they began. Anxiety may be experienced prior to an attack, followed by relief and relaxation afterwards, leading some to speculate that psychogenic seizures may occur as a direct response to stress to relieve tension. Afterwards, patients usually have a vague recollection of the seizure, without the usual postseizure symptoms of drowsiness and depression.

Differentiating between psychogenic and epileptic seizures is difficult. Epileptic seizures and pseudoseizures are distinguishable by both their nature and their symptoms. Research indicates that, in 20% to 30% of cases, physicians who specialize in the diagnosis and treatment of epilepsy are incorrect in attempting to distinguish one from the other. Epileptic seizures are caused by a change in how the brain cells send electrical signals to each other, whereas pseudoseizures are triggered by a conscious or unconscious desire for more care and attention. Thus, measuring brain activity with an EEG and video telemetry is important for distinguishing epileptic from pseudoseizures. Also, pseudoseizures often lack the exhaustion, confusion, and nausea that are associated with epileptic seizure activity. It is important to remember that psychogenic seizures can occur in individuals who also experience epileptic seizures.

The appropriate treatment for pseudoseizures is to calm the person and start him or her breathing at a normal rate. Treatment should also involve investigating the mental and emotional factors that led to the psuedoseizure. Medications are ineffective in the treatment of this disorder. Patients are usually referred for psychotherapy. Because the vast majority of psychogenic seizures involve intrapersonal and interpersonal dynamics as well as behavioral manifestations, focused psychotherapy, including behavioral interventions, is usually indicated.

Hypertension

Cardiovascular diseases such as *hypertension*—that is, high blood pressure, heart disease, and stroke—are the cause of almost 1 million deaths in the United States each year. They are the leading cause of death among both men and women and across all racial and ethnic groups. About 58 million Americans live with some form of the disease. In 1999 alone, cardiovascular diseases cost the nation an estimated $287 billion in health care expenditures and lost productivity, and this burden is growing as the population ages. Three health behaviors—cigarette smoking, lack of physical activity, and poor nutrition—are major risk factors for the cardiovascular diseases. This section focuses primarily on hypertension.

Currently, approximately 25% of the world's adult population is hypertensive. Two thirds of Americans over the age of 60 have elevated blood pressures. More than 43 million individuals in the United States have hypertension, but less than one third achieves an adequate level of blood pressure control, due in part to the fact that self-management of blood pressure control is not yet widely practiced. Blood pressure is extremely variable over time and is influenced by physical activity as well as mental stress. For this reason, frequent measurement often yields artificially high readings, that is, the so-called *white coat effect*. A growing body of research indicates that tight blood pressure control improves the cardiovascular and microvascular complications of diabetes. Although the current gold standard for 24-hour blood pressure is ambulatory monitoring, it is too expensive to offer to large groups, such as those with Type 2 diabetes.

Because the association between blood pressure and cardiovascular risk is continuous, there is no threshold above which the risk suddenly increases. Until further trials document the predictive value of blood pressure levels to target organ damage, 135/85 is considered the upper limit of normal. Office blood pressure measurement by a physician with a mercury sphygmomanometer remains the standard because its relationship with cardiovascular prognosis has been demonstrated. Although blood pressure units available for home measurement are not as accurate as office blood pressure instruments, it is more important that patients do daily monitoring of their blood pressure, particularly if it is in the high range.

Given that hypertension is a silent disease, overt symptoms are rarely experienced compared with other chronic diseases. Therefore, self-management is quite important. Current self-management programs focus on home blood pressure monitoring with a protocol in which individuals adjust their own drug therapy if readings consistently exceed their established limits.

Exercise, relaxation strategies, and diet modification are standard elements of these protocols.

Irritable Bowel Syndrome

IBS is a disorder that interferes with the normal functions of the large intestine, that is, colon. It is characterized by the following symptoms: crampy abdominal pain, bloating, constipation, and diarrhea. IBS is much more common than most think; it is the second-leading cause of absenteeism from work and school, after the common cold. One in five Americans experience IBS, making it one of the most commonly diagnosed disorders today. It occurs more often in women than in men, and it usually begins around age 20. Individuals with IBS appear to have colons that are more sensitive and react to things that might not bother other people, such as stress, large meals, gas, medicines, certain foods, caffeine, or alcohol.

Although IBS engenders considerable discomfort and distress, it does not permanently damage the intestines or lead to cancer or intestinal bleeding, and it is not related to Crohn's disease or ulcerative colitis. Most individuals can control their symptoms with diet, stress management, and medications prescribed by their physician. Nevertheless, for some individuals, IBS can be disabling in that affected individuals may be unable to work, go to social events, or travel even short distances.

The cause of IBS is unknown. Research suggests that those with IBS seem to have a heightened colon sensitivity and reactivity, particularly to certain foods and stress. Some evidence indicates that the immune system is also involved. IBS symptoms appear to result from abnormal motility of the colon, that is, the contraction of the colon muscles and the movement of its contents. The *epithelial lining* of the colon regulates the passage of fluids in and out of the colon. In IBS, the epithelium appears to work properly, but fast movement of the colon's contents can overcome its absorptive capacity. The result is too much fluid in the stool. In other individuals, colonic movement is too slow, too much fluid is absorbed, and constipation develops.

The colon responds strongly to stimuli such as foods and stress. However, in those with IBS, stress and emotions can strongly affect the colon. The colon may contract too much or too little or may absorb too much or too little water. The following have been associated with a worsening of IBS symptoms: large meals; bloating from gas in the colon; medicines; wheat, rye, barley, chocolate, milk products, and alcohol; drinks with caffeine, such as coffee, tea, and soft drinks; and stress, conflict, and emotional upsets. Research has determined that women with IBS tend to have more symptoms during their menstrual periods, suggesting that reproductive hormones can exacerbate IBS problems.

Abdominal pain or discomfort in association with bowel dysfunction is the main symptom of IBS, but symptoms vary from person to person. Some experience constipation, others diarrhea, and still others alternating constipation and diarrhea. Some also experience bloating and the sensation of pressure inside the abdomen. Others report a crampy urge to move their bowels but cannot do so or pass mucus with their bowel movements. It is important to note that bleeding, fever, weight loss, and persistent severe pain are never symptoms of IBS and may indicate other problems, such as inflammation or rarely, cancer.

IBS is generally diagnosed on the basis of a complete medical history that includes a careful description of symptoms and a physical examination. No particular test is specific for IBS; however, diagnostic tests may be performed to rule out other diseases, such as Crohn's and ulcerative colitis. These tests may include stool or blood tests, x-rays, or endoscopy (viewing the colon through a flexible tube inserted through the anus). If these tests are all negative, a diagnosis of IBS may be based entirely on history and symptoms, that is, the intensity and duration of abdominal pain during the past year, the nature and quality of the pain in relation to bowel function, and bowel frequency and stool consistency. Diagnostic criteria for this disorder include abdominal pain or discomfort for at least 12 weeks out of the previous 12 months, and the pain or discomfort must have two of the following three features: (a) It is relieved by having a bowel movement; (b) when it starts, there is a change in how often the person has a bowel movement; and (c) when it starts, there is a change in the form of the stool or the way it looks.

Currently, no cure is available for IBS, but many options are available to treat the symptoms. Among these is self-management, which, when based on the optimal combination of medication, diet, health counseling, and support, can effectively control symptoms. Medications are an important part of relieving symptoms. A doctor may suggest fiber supplements or occasional laxatives for constipation, as well as medicines to decrease diarrhea, tranquilizers to calm the patient, or drugs that control colon muscle spasms to reduce abdominal pain. Antidepressants may also relieve some symptoms. Medications available to treat IBS specifically are the following: Lotronex for women with severe IBS who have not responded to conventional therapy and whose primary symptom is diarrhea, and Zelnorm for the short-term treatment of women with IBS whose primary symptom is constipation. Laxatives can be habit forming if they are not used carefully or are used too frequently.

Stress stimulates colon spasms in IBS. The colon has a vast supply of nerves that control its normal rhythmic contractions and cause abdominal discomfort at stressful times, resulting in cramps or "butterflies." In IBS, the colon is often overly responsive to even slight conflict or stress. Some evidence suggests that IBS is affected by the immune system, and the immune system is also affected by stress. Thus, stress management is an essential strategy for managing IBS. Stress management comprises relaxation training and relaxation therapies, meditation, regular exercise such as walking or yoga, adequate sleep, health counseling, and, when indicated, psychotherapy. Psychotherapeutic strategies, including brief psychodynamic therapy, cognitive–behavioral therapy (CBT), and hypnotherapy, have been used successfully with IBS (Blanchard, 2001).

Careful eating can reduce IBS symptoms. Preferred diets are low in fat and high in carbohydrates, such as pasta, rice, whole-grain breads and cereals, fruits, and vegetables. Keeping a journal of offending foods and consultation with a dietitian or nutritionist can be helpful. Often, dietary fiber can lessen IBS symptoms, particularly constipation, but may not help pain or diarrhea. High-fiber diets keep the colon mildly distended, which may help prevent spasms. Some forms of fiber also keep water in the stool, thereby preventing hard stools that are difficult to pass. Accordingly, diets with sufficient fiber to produce soft, painless bowel movements are routinely prescribed. Although high-fiber diets may cause gas and bloating, these symptoms often remit within a few weeks as the gastrointestinal system adjusts. Sufficient water intake is also important. Eating smaller meals more often or eating smaller portions should help IBS symptoms because large meals can cause cramping and diarrhea.

Systemic Lupus Erythematosus

SLE is an autoimmune disease, that is, a disease in which the immune system turns against parts of the body it is designed to protect. The result is inflammation and tissue damage. SLE can affect various body systems, including the joints, skin, kidneys, heart, lungs, blood vessels, and brain. SLE is characterized by periods of exacerbation of symptoms, called *flares*, and periods of remission. At present, there is no cure for SLE. However, it can be effectively treated and managed, and most individuals with the disease can lead active, healthy lives. Most SLE patients (78%) reported that they are coping well with their illness. Pain (65%), lifestyle changes (61%), and emotional problems associated with the illness (50%) were reported as the most difficult factors for coping with SLE. With appropriate medical care and self-management, 80% to 90% of those with SLE can expect to live a normal life span.

SLE can occur at any age and in either sex. Nine out of ten people with lupus are women. During the childbearing years, SLE is found in women 10 to 15 times more frequently than in men. SLE is 3 times more common in African American women than in Caucasian women and is more common in women of Hispanic, Asian, or Native American descent. It is interesting to note that SLE can run in families, but the risk is rather low.

Besides SLE, three other types of lupus are recognized: *discoid lupus erythematosus*, a chronic skin disorder in which a red, raised rash appears on the face, scalp, or elsewhere; *subacute cutaneous lupus erythematosus*, a milder disease characterized by skin lesions that appear on parts of the body exposed to sun; and *drug-induced lupus*, which is caused by medications and which presents with symptoms similar to SLE. The Lupus Foundation of America estimates that approximately 1,500,000 Americans have a type of lupus, with over 70% having SLE.

SLE is a complex disease, and its cause is unknown. It is likely that a combination of genetic, environmental, and possibly hormonal factors work together to cause the disease. Although to date no specific "SLE gene" has been identified, studies suggest that several different genes may be involved in determining an individual's likelihood for developing the disease, which tissues and organs will be affected, and the severity of disease. It is believed that certain factors trigger SLE, such as stress, sunlight, certain drugs, and viruses. It is likely that a combination of factors is involved in the expression of the disease.

Every individual with SLE has slightly different symptoms, which can range from mild to severe and may come and go over time. Nevertheless, there are common symptoms that characterize this condition: painful or swollen joints (i.e., arthritis); unexplained fever; extreme fatigue; a characteristic red skin rash across the nose and cheeks, that is, the so-called *butterfly rash* or *malar rash*; chest pain on deep breathing; unusual loss of hair; pale or purple fingers or toes from cold or stress, that is, *Raynaud's phenomenon*; sensitivity to the sun; swelling in the legs or around the eyes; mouth ulcers; swollen glands; and extreme fatigue. Some experience headaches, dizziness, depression, confusion, or seizures. New symptoms may continue to appear years after the initial diagnosis, and different symptoms can occur at different times.

A number of systems in the body also can be affected by SLE. Inflammation of the kidneys (i.e., *nephritis*) can impair their ability to get rid of waste products and other toxins from the body effectively. Some develop *pleuritis*, an inflammation of the lining of the chest cavity that causes chest pain, particularly with breathing. They may also get pneumonia. SLE can affect the brain or central nervous system, causing headaches, dizziness, memory disturbances, vision problems, seizures, stroke, or changes in behavior. Blood vessels may become inflamed (i.e., *vasculitis*), affecting the way blood circulates through the body. The inflammation may be mild and may not require treatment or may be severe and require immediate attention. Some may develop anemia; *leukopenia*, that is, a decreased number of white blood cells; or *thrombocytopenia*, that is, a decrease in the number of platelets in the blood, which assist in clotting. Others may have an increased risk for blood clots. In others, inflammation can occur in the heart itself, that is, *myocarditis* or *endocarditis*, or the membrane that surrounds it, that is, *pericarditis*, causing chest pains or other symptoms. SLE can also increase the risk of *atherosclerosis*, that is, hardening of the arteries.

Diagnosing SLE is often difficult, and it may take months or even years for a correct diagnosis to be made and confirmed. Reaching a diagnosis may take time as new symptoms appear. Unfortunately, no single test can confirm the diagnosis. The most useful tests such as the antinuclear antibody

(ANA), anti-DNA, anti-Sm, anti-RNP, anti-Ro (SSA), and anti-La (SSB) tests identify certain autoantibodies.

The diagnosis and treatment of SLE is typically a collaborative effort between the patient and several types of health care clinicians: family physicians or internists, rheumatologists, clinical immunologists, nephrologists, hematologists, dermatologists, and neurologists, as well as nurses, psychologists, mental health counselors, and social workers. The range and effectiveness of treatments for SLE have increased dramatically, giving clinicians more choices in managing the disease. It is important for the patient to work closely with clinicians and to take an active role in self-managing the disease. Once SLE has been diagnosed, the physician will develop a treatment plan tailored to the severity of the disorder as well as the patient's age, sex, health, symptoms, and lifestyle. Because of the variability of SLE and its response to interventions, the treatment plan is likely to change over time. There is no permanent cure for SLE. The goal of treatment is to relieve symptoms and protect organs by decreasing inflammation and the level of autoimmune activity in the body. Many with mild symptoms may need little or no treatment or only intermittent courses of anti-inflammatory medications. Those with more serious presentations, that is, damage to internal organs, may require a rigorous medication regimen to suppress the overactive immune system.

There are currently several conventional medical treatments for SLE. They are prescribed on the basis of the type and severity of symptoms. For those with joint or chest pain or fever, anti-inflammatory drugs, that is, NSAIDs, such as ibuprofen and naproxen, may be used alone or in combination with other drugs to control pain, swelling, and fever. Antimalarials, such as hydroxychloroquine (Plaquenil), are another type of drug commonly used to treat SLE. Although originally used to treat malaria, they have been found useful for SLE. The mainstay of SLE treatment involves the use of corticosteroid hormones, such as prednisone (Deltasone), hydrocortisone, methylprednisolone (Medrol), and dexamethasone (Decadron, Hexadrol). Corticosteroids work by rapidly suppressing inflammation and can be given orally, in creams applied to the skin, or by injection. For some individuals whose kidneys or central nervous systems are affected by SLE, an immunosuppressive drug, such as cyclophosphamide (Cytoxan) and mycophenolate mofetil (CellCept), may be used. These drugs effectively dampen the overactive immune system by blocking the production of immune cells. In some patients, methotrexate (Folex, Mexate, Rheumatrex), a disease-modifying antirheumatic drug, may be used to help control the disease.

Besides medication, several environmental and psychosocial interventions are involved in the treatment process and are mainstays of self-management. Environmental factors that trigger or exacerbate SLE include UV light, particularly sunlight; diet; and bacterial and viral infections. Interventions usually involve limiting or eliminating exposure to these factors (Digeronimo, 2002). For instance, most SLE patients soon learn that avoiding exposure to the midday sun is essential to their well-being. Psychosocial interventions include relaxation techniques and CBT. Because stress is both a trigger of and a response to SLE, effectively managing it is a key goal of self-management. Relaxation techniques include deep breathing, mental imagery, progressive muscle relaxation, and biofeedback.

CBT can be particularly useful in dealing with denial of the illness, as well as in changing negative thinking, the excessive use of drugs, the avoidance of activity, and dependence on others. CBT can foster and reward the opposites of these thoughts, that is, responsibility, independence, activity, and a desire to free oneself from the constraints of SLE rather than be bound by it. CBT can help patients attend to what they think and say about their illness and can provide a method of redirecting their thinking in a positive direction so that they can recognize their self-talk and attitudes and identify beliefs that make it more difficult for them to live with this chronic condition (Digeronimo, 2002). As with other chronic illnesses, it is essential to self-management that patients understand the relationship between the way they think about their health and the way they feel, as reflected in their energy level, their attitudes, their moods, and their behavior.

Lately, alternative and complementary medical treatments have become popular in the treatment of SLE, both because of the cost of conventional medications and their potential for serious side effects. Alternative treatment approaches include special diets, nutritional supplements, fish oils, ointments and creams, chiropractic treatment, and homeopathy. Although some of these treatment approaches have been associated with symptomatic or psychosocial benefits, there is little or no research to date that shows that they affect the disease process or prevent organ damage. Some alternative or complementary approaches may help the patient cope with or reduce some of the stress associated with living with a chronic illness. If the doctor feels the approach has value and will not be harmful, it can be incorporated into the patient's treatment plan. However, it is important not to neglect regular health care or treatment of serious symptoms.

CONCLUDING NOTE

Psychologically trained clinicians working with chronic illness must acquire some basic knowledge of specific chronic diseases and the chronic disease processes, but it is even more important that such clinicians understand how chronic disease processes impact personality; how social and cultural aspects influence the experience of the disease; and how personality, culture, and social factors impact the disease process. Unlike physicians, these clinicians do not need the exact knowledge and understanding of pathophysiological processes but will be well served by a general understanding of pathological processes for the specific disease conditions with which they are working. This chapter provided basic information on 10 common chronic medical illnesses.

Additional information can be accessed from textbooks of medicine, book chapters, and articles in professional journals, as well as Internet sites of the various National Institutes of Health. These sites contain accurate and up-to-date information on the diagnosis and treatment of basically all acute and chronic medical conditions. Other sources of information include other health care providers, particularly the physician of record. Because treating patients with chronic illness typically involves some collaboration with medical and health care professionals, psychologists and therapists will usually find that these medical professionals will share information about the patient's condition, the disease process, and the diagnostic and treatment regimen. In my experience, knowledge sharing is not uncommon among professionals. Accordingly, medical personnel will be receptive to discussing the medical aspects of cases with psychologists and other mental health professionals, just as they may want to learn from psychologists and other mental health professionals about how personality and psychological dynamics impact disease processes.

4

PERSONALITY AND CHRONIC ILLNESS

In chapter 2, personality was characterized as a key factor in both the psychosocial model and the biopsychosocial model of chronic illness. *Personality style* is used in this chapter to describe the unique characteristics of an individual's personality. This term can be defined as an individual's enduring pattern of thinking, feeling, behaving, and relating to the environment in a consistent manner and in various social contexts (Sperry, 2003a). A *personality disorder* is present when a personality style becomes sufficiently inflexible and maladaptive and causes significant impairment in occupational or social functioning or when it results in great subjective distress. A personality disorder indicates the existence of a long-standing maladaptive pattern of attitudes and behaviors of the way an individual relates to, perceives, and thinks about the environment and him- or herself and that is of sufficient severity to cause either significant impairment in adaptive functioning or subjective distress. Characteristically, those with personality disorders have difficulty taking responsibility for their behavior and cooperating with others. Although everyone exhibits a characteristic personality style, not all manifest a personality disorder (Sperry, 2003a).

In health care situations, this means that personality-disordered clients are a challenge to health care personnel with regard to engagement in the treatment process, that is, keeping appointments, following treatment recommendations, and relating to others, particularly health care professionals. The presence of a personality disorder invariably complicates the treatment process in clients with chronic illness. Six personality styles are commonly seen in those with chronic illness. These are as follows: compulsive personality, histrionic personality, dependent personality, avoidant personality, narcissistic personality, and borderline personality (Sperry, 1999b; Stone, 1993).

Each of these six personality styles or disorders is described in terms of health-related dynamics that reflect the uniqueness of their underlying personality dynamics, their illness representation, and their likely response to clinicians and the treatment process. Because diabetes is such a widely prevalent chronic disease today, the health dynamics of each of the personality styles are illustrated with regard to diabetes. The interested reader can find an extended description of these personality styles in Sperry (2003a) and their characteristic health dynamics in Harper (2003).

COMPULSIVE PERSONALITY

People with a compulsive personality can be recognized behavior and interpersonal styles, cognitive style, and emotional style. Their behavior is characterized by perfectionism. Individuals with this disorder are likely to be workaholics. In addition to exhibiting dependability, they tend to be stubborn and possessive. They, like people with passive–aggressive disorder, can be indecisive and procrastinating. Interpersonally, these individuals are exquisitely conscious of social rank and status and modify their behavior accordingly. That is, they tend to be deferential and obsequious to superiors and haughty and autocratic to subordinates and peers. They can be doggedly insistent that others do things their way, without an appreciation or awareness of how others react to this insistence. At their best, they are polite and loyal to the organizations and ideals they espouse.

Their thinking style can be characterized as constricted and rule based. They have difficulty establishing priorities and perspective. They are "detail" people and often lose sight of the larger project. In other words, they "can't see the forest for the trees." Their indecisiveness and doubts make decision making difficult. Their mental inflexibility is matched by their nonsuggestible and unimaginative style, suggesting that they have a restricted fantasy life. Like individuals who are passive–aggressive, those who are compulsive have conflicts between assertiveness and defiance, and pleasing and obedience.

Their emotional style is characterized as grim and cheerless. They have difficulty with the expression of intimate feelings such as warmth and tenderness. They tend to avoid the "softer" feelings, although they may express anger, frustration, and irritability quite freely. This grim, feeling-avoidant demeanor shows itself in stilted, stiff relationship behaviors (Sperry, 2003a).

Developmental and Etiological Features

The biopsychosocial formulation that follows may be helpful in understanding how this style or disorder is likely to have developed. Biologically, these individuals were likely to have exhibited an anhedonic temperament as an infant (Millon, 1981). Firstborn children have a greater propensity for developing a compulsive style than other siblings.

Psychologically, these individuals view themselves, others, the world, and life's purpose in terms of the following themes. They view themselves with some variant of the theme "I'm responsible if something goes wrong, so I have to be reliable, competent, and righteous." Their worldview is some variant of the theme "Life is unpredictable and expects too much." As such, they are likely to conclude, "Therefore, be in control, right, and proper at all times."

Socially, predictable patterns of parenting and environmental conditioning are noted for this personality. The parenting style they experienced could be characterized as both consistent and overcontrolled. As children, they were trained to be overly responsible for their actions and to feel guilty and worthless if they were not obedient, achievement oriented, or "good." The parental injunction to which they were most likely exposed was "You must do and be better to be worthwhile."

This compulsive pattern is confirmed, reinforced, and perpetuated by the following individual and systems factors: exceedingly high expectations plus harshly rigid behavior and beliefs, along with a tendency to be self-critical, leading to rigid rule-based behavior and avoidance of social, professional, and moral unacceptability. This in turn further reconfirms the harshly rigid behaviors and beliefs of this personality style (Sperry, 2003a).

Health-Related Dynamics

Individuals with a compulsive personality represent the conscientious, virtuous patient with considerable respect for authority. Under ordinary circumstances, the patient–clinician relationship will be especially satisfying for people with this personality style. It is not surprising that the exception is when their chronic illness is perceived as a threat. Such a threat arises when no cure is available or there is no immediate treatment plan. Uncertainty generates anxiety, and they will press clinicians for specifics and clarity, which often are not possible. In turn, the clinician may become frustrated and project anger in reaction to these anxious demands. Because of their conflicts concerning dependency needs, help seeking and the acceptance and use of social support tends to be difficult for them to accept. Because their pattern has been to give rather than to receive, patients with a compulsive personality are often not accustomed to reciprocating.

Patients with a compulsive style tend to be sensitizers rather than re-pressors. Accordingly, they will benefit from information that provides them with predictability. However, when illness courses do not follow predicted paths or when there are unexpected adverse events, these patients can experience a loss of control that could be overwhelming for them. Monitoring their anxiety level when distressing information is imparted concerning the probable course of their illness and its treatment is important to ensuring that these patients do not become overwhelmed with the response to their questions and generate more information than they can reasonably handle. It is also important that the diagnosis of their chronic disease occur as early as possible. Otherwise clinicians should expect that these patients will respond by reporting baffling and vague symptoms or even anxiety-generated false alarms, which are bothersome to clinicians.

Illness representations by patients with a compulsive personality are often characterized by a mix of anxiety-ridden, overideational concerns and overly concrete conceptions that are centered on fears of loss of mastery and control. Accordingly, they attempt to develop self-reassuring schemas or frantically seek alternative medicine explanations to protect themselves from what medical science can only partially address. This will lead to rigid calm and inflexible adherence to alternative medical treatment objectives as they attempt to manage their treatment, possibly to the detriment of their own health and almost always to the detriment of their relationship with their original clinicians and treatment teams. Given their conflicted dependency, their use of health care resources varies from discomfort to fruitless overuse in their quest to achieve an illusion of control where none may be possible. Secondary gain for these patients typically involves relief from burdensome responsibility and from fears of failure. It may also legitimatize a repressed longing to being cared for by others (Harper, 2003).

Clinicians not only can help these patients tremendously but also can help themselves to the extent that they recognize that the patients do experience relief and a sense of personal control and mastery from medical explanations and information sharing, particularly in the face of unexpected developments, and to the extent that they are willing to put up with repetitive, annoying questions and assurance seeking. Such clinician efforts do much to restore the defenses of these patients so that they more effectively cope and participate as the good patients they wish to be.

The need for control and mastery by people who have a compulsive style makes them interpersonally trying to clinicians, particularly when these patients can become overinvolved with their care, monitor clinicians' activities, ask endless and repetitive questions, and even seek to take over their own care. In some instances, they make adjustments to their medications on the basis of their idiosyncratic understanding because of the unpleasant side effects or because of specific main effects—for example, pain relief—they wish to obtain. When they are caught engaging in such behavior, they may be predictably embarrassed but also remain anxious unless they are reassured that everything is being done to help them. When their efforts at autonomy, however injudicious, are thwarted, they may experience unrecognized feelings of resentment. Although their presentation will be that of a conscientious, obedient patient, if the treatment course or drug effects take an unusual turn, they can be expected to meddle in their treatment when it is not going the way they expect or silently demand.

Clinicians can precipitate an interpersonal crisis if they unwittingly accuse such patients of wrongdoing or meddling. This is because these patients view themselves as being virtuous, helpful, and conscientious. If mistaken, the clinician has wrongly conveyed a lack of confidence in the patient, which undermines his or her sense of being an important part of the treatment process.

Because such individuals are oriented toward others, their functioning during times of illness will be to seek authority outside themselves for ways in which to respond, rather than to focus on their work with clinicians. This has to do with poorly recognized conflicts and feelings stemming from the stress of being removed from their constricted comfort zones.

When an unfavorable illness course is anticipated or emerges from the chronic disease process, these patients need assistance in processing the implications of such changes in the way they represent their illness to themselves. This is best accomplished in a judicious fashion, because preserving their compulsive defenses is a key treatment goal, assuming that those defenses do not impede any necessary emotional work from eventually taking place. The clinician is advised to remain sensitive to where the patient with obsessive–compulsive personality disorder is emotionally and to offer counseling for depressive or anxiety symptoms as they develop. Arguably, the timing of the introduction of psychotherapy is critical. Premature introduction has been known to preempt their own efforts to cope and could unnecessarily foster regression into a helpless dependency rather than stabilize them emotionally (Harper, 2003).

The Experience of Diabetes

Of all the personality styles, the compulsive personality style seems to be best suited for dealing with a chronic illness like diabetes, an illness requiring lifelong self-monitoring, discipline, self-denial, and self-regulation. Provided that diabetic self-care measures can be integrated into the daily routines and health patterns of the patient with a compulsive personality, they will become part of their rigid mode of functioning. Difficulties that do arise in the treatment process are more likely to emerge early in the treatment course rather than later. Specifically, problems are noted in initially establishing health behavior changes. If the diabetic condition is diagnosed in older individuals whose routines are already deeply ingrained and who may have strong appetites that must be curbed, such as for sugar, alcohol, caffeine, and nicotine, such health behavior changes pit unhealthy, but automatic, routines and habits against the good intentions of the individual with a compulsive personality to preserve his or her health and conform to medical recommendations.

Because diabetes is a lifelong condition with serious consequences for nonadherence, there are many incentives for these individuals to reduce their risk behaviors. It is important that clinicians recognize the unique dynamics of the compulsive personality style and tailor their response to patients' efforts to establish and maintain the requisite health behaviors. Thus, being too harsh in evaluating early deviations from the treatment plan as these individuals struggle to conform can be counterproductive. Such harshness may actually intensify their preoccupation with punishment, leading to greater rigidity in their mode of coping. Furthermore, if their experience of shame is too intense, their determined efforts to change may be replaced with fear and avoidance behaviors, which are likely to result in their withholding or concealing evidence of nonadherence. It is not surprising that this will be accompanied by nonproductive guilt, self-recrimination, and a distancing of themselves from health care providers. For this reason, it is essential to communicate an accepting, supportive attitude toward these patients, recognizing their struggles and conflicts, while conveying confidence that they are doing enough to manage their illness, despite occasional lapses (Harper, 2003).

HISTRIONIC PERSONALITY

The clinical presentation of the histrionic personality can be characterized with the following behavioral and interpersonal styles, thinking style, and feeling style. The behavioral style is characterized as charming, dramatic, and expressive, while also being demanding, self-indulgent, and inconsiderate. Persistent attention seeking, mood lability, capriciousness, and superficiality further characterize the behavior of individuals with a histrionic style. Interpersonally, these individuals tend to be exhibitionistic and flirtatious in their manner, with attention seeking and manipulativeness being prominent.

The thinking or cognitive style of this personality can be characterized as impulsive and thematic, rather than analytical, precise, and field independent. In short, their tendency is to be nonanalytic, vague, and field dependent. They are easily suggestible and rely heavily on hunches and intuition. They avoid awareness of their own hidden dependency and other self-knowledge and tend to be "other directed" with respect to the need for approval from others. Therefore, they can easily dissociate their "real" or inner self from their "public" or outer self. Their emotional or affective style is characterized by exaggerated emotional displays and excitability, including irrational outbursts and temper tantrums. Although they are constantly seeking reassurance that they are loved, they respond with only superficial warmth and charm and are generally emotionally shallow. Finally, they are exceedingly rejection sensitive (Sperry, 2003a).

Development and Etiological Features

The following biopsychosocial formulation may be helpful in understanding how the histrionic personality develops. Biologically and temperamentally, the histrionic personality appears to be quite different from the dependent personality. Unlike the dependent personality, the histrionic personality is characterized by a high energy level and emotional and autonomic reactivity. Millon and Everly (1985) noted that adults who are histrionic tended to display a high degree of emotional lability and responsiveness in their infancy and early childhood. Their temperament, then, can be characterized as hyperresponsive and externally oriented for gratification. Psychologically, this style or disorder holds a characteristic self-view, worldview, and life goal. The self-view of the person with a histrionic personality is some variant of the theme "I am sensitive and everyone should admire and approve of me." The worldview is some variant of "Life makes me nervous, so I am entitled to special care and consideration." Their life goal is some variant of the theme "Therefore, play to the audience, and have fun, fun, fun."

In addition to biological and psychological factors, social factors, such as parenting style and injunction, and family and environmental factors, influence the development of the histrionic personality style. The parental injunction for the histrionic personality style involves reciprocity: "I'll give you attention if you do X." A parenting style that involves minimal or inconsistent discipline helps ensure and reinforce the histrionic pattern. The child who is histrionic is likely to grow up with at least one parent who is manipulative or histrionic, who reinforces the child's histrionic and attention-seeking behavior. Finally, the following sequence of self and system perpetuants are likely to be seen in the person with a histrionic personality disorder: denial of one's real or inner self; a preoccupation with externals; the need for excitement and attention seeking, which leads to a superficial charm and interpersonal presence; and the need for external approval. This, in turn, further reinforces the dissociation and denial of the real or inner self from the public self, and the cycle continues (Sperry, 2003a).

Health-Related Dynamics

The egocentric, attention-seeking nature of those with a histrionic personality in health care settings makes them highly visible and even at times entertaining for clinicians. This attention-seeking manner may wear thin during intense periods of the treatment process. Clinicians will observe how these individuals manipulate social situations to serve their need for attention. When chronic disease diagnosis is delayed in such patients, it may result from a clinician's loss of sensitivity to them after experiencing several false alarms and frequently confusing arrays of patient symptoms and complaints. Adherence to treatment regimens can also be erratic, given their flighty nature, along with their reluctance to assume responsibility for their care. The way in which they represent their illness and their symptomatic complaints typically assumes dramatic forms and proportions in their effort to secure an audience and support their egocentric attention needs. However, if a clinician can remain tolerant and meets some of their interpersonal needs, these individuals can remain reasonably engaged in the treatment process, unlike many other personality styles that are at risk for dropping out of treatment except when confronted with serious medical concerns.

It is noteworthy that for certain medical conditions, the vanity and social consciousness of these patients is a primary motivating factor in early disease detection. For instance, the threat of disfiguring breast or skin cancer or debilitating heart disease may strike sufficient fear to be highly vigilant of early warning signs in individuals with a histrionic personality who are at high risk for such conditions. However, less visible conditions, such as hypertension, often escape their attention unless unpleasant symptoms, such as headache or dizziness, are present.

When a chronic condition is diagnosed, these patients tend to incorporate it into their interpersonal style repertoire, a repertoire characterized by dramatization, particularly with regard to the relationship with their clinicians. Provided that they are fashionable to display to family, friends, and even strangers, the symptoms associated with their condition can also serve an attention-seeking function. Conversion and dissociation can also characterize this histrionic style. Because clinicians rely on symptoms to gauge disease progression, response to treatment, and other aspects of the chronic condition, this dissociation from the underlying physiological process is often problematic and frustrating for clinicians. In the course of doing a review of disease-related symptoms, the clinician can unwittingly facilitate the conversion reaction process because the histrionic personality style is highly suggestible and so is vulnerable to conversion and dissociation. Even a true manifestation of disease-related symptoms can serve as a model for later pseudosymptomatic episodes. Even though these patients have a long history of false alarms, wasted clinic visits, and exhausted family caretakers, their "cried-wolf" pattern does not in any way immunize them against the emergence of a potentially debilitating disease at some time or other. Thus, patience is the byword in working with this personality type. In terms of secondary gain considerations, attention seeking is the most likely outcome of symptom magnification. Nevertheless, avoidance of conflict and relinquishment of unwanted responsibilities are other sources of secondary gain (Harper, 2003).

Efforts to increase independence and self-mastery in these patients may be doomed to frustration or failure if the clinician fails to recognize their superficial interpersonal needs. Any intervention that serves to reduce contact and distance them from clinicians runs counter to their basic strategy. Thus, clinician efforts or recommendations to increase independence will be ignored unless self-mastery serves to gain social attention for them. For example, it can be advantageous to have a patient promise to call at a fixed or scheduled time that is convenient for the clinician to report how she or he is doing when asymptomatic. Therapeutic tactics such as this serve to reduce erroneous symptom reporting while addressing the social demand that is an inescapable, inherent part of the clinician–patient relationship for these patients.

Patient interactions with clinicians is characterized by a supercilious presentation, wherein, for each item of relevant medical or therapeutic information, the clinician will have to listen to and acknowledge several lengthy details of often irrelevant personal or interpersonal information. Unfortunately, this is an essential and necessary quid pro quo; that is, meaningful information is exchanged for interpersonal attention and acknowledgment. When clinicians communicate their annoyance with such supercilious behavior in a serious medical context, it can distract or upset these patients, who may respond by becoming more frantic or exaggerated in their symptomatic presentation aimed at capturing the clinicians' attention. However, warmly attending to such individuals for a reasonable period of time may satisfy their need for interaction and may paradoxically gain the clinician's credibility for more serious discussion and the transmission of important, authoritative health information.

The manner in which individuals with a histrionic personality represent their illness tends to be emotionally charged and dramatic, and it serves to draw attention to themselves. Simply providing accurate, objective information concerning a disease process for these individuals does not necessary engender an accurate understanding of their condition. Rather, the clinician's information can be transformed in some particular fashion peculiar to the patient. Accurate representation may require review and clarification with the patient, who may still distort the information initially, although the nature of the distortion can be quite informative for the clinician. The more concrete the illness representation information can be made and linked to the patient's specific experience and need for adherence behavior, the more likely there will be treatment adherence. Although for some individuals, accurate information about a disease process can constitute a reassuring sense of control, this is rarely important for individuals with a histrionic style. Rather, what is important is how the information and behavioral expectations are related to the patient's sense of relationship with the clinician. It is only such relational information that is deemed important to this type of patient.

The treatment of patients with a histrionic personality disorder must, out of necessity, address their impulsivity, fickle social behavior, and overreactivity to situations, particularly those of a negative nature. Cognitive–behavioral therapy appears to be quite helpful in addressing their lack of reflectivity and tendency to disassociate when faced with conflicts and other stressors. Such behavior patterns prevent them from developing a true sense of continuity and from learning new adaptive behavior patterns. Assuming that these individuals are sufficiently motivated to engage in behavior change, focused problem-oriented psychotherapeutic interventions can be quite effective. Assertiveness training can be a powerful tactic and can substitute for seductive behavior and attention-seeking activity because it helps reduce their conflict avoiding tendencies. In addition, relaxation training can be useful in decreasing arousal level, excitability, and tendency to somatize, all of which are characteristics of this personality type (Harper, 2003).

The Experience of Diabetes

Childhood or adolescent Type 1 diabetes, although typically more severe and brittle than Type 2 diabetes, provides young individuals the opportunity to develop critical self-management skills using blood sugar monitoring and insulin injections. Self-management of early-onset diabetes establishes habit patterns that are quite challenging for those with a later life onset of this chronic disease. It is a challenge that is particularly difficult for individuals who are histrionic to meet successfully, given their rather fragmented, undisciplined existence. Thus, for adults with a histrionic personality who are diagnosed with Type 2 diabetes, the challenge of developing appropriate health habits and a disciplined daily regimen of regulating their blood sugar levels, calculating calories, and evaluating food choices, especially when dining out, can be overwhelming. These patients inevitably require longer and more varied training to achieve sufficient proficiency in disease management applicable to their particular circumstances. Often it is useful to introduce a social dimension in this training, given the gregarious interpersonal nature of this personality type. It is not surprising that skill-training groups and dining-out groups are popular and effective with these individuals.

Extreme blood sugar levels, that is, hypoglycemia or hyperglycemia, can be a potentially serious weapon in the hands of individuals with a strong need for attention. Individuals who are histrionic have been known to demand attention and caretaking by precipitating a diabetic crisis, particularly when they believe a valued relationship is being threatened. Furthermore, their natural excitability can also generate stress-related hormonal changes. In the aftermath of crises of this type, clinicians may conclude that this action involved deliberate nonadherence and justifies their censure or disapproval. Predictably, the individual with a histrionic style will react with frenetic activity to seek social assurance, engaging in behavior that may ultimately undermine previous efforts to develop stable disease control routines. Clinicians would do well to help these patients process the situation and find alternative and less medically risky solutions (Harper, 2003).

DEPENDENT PERSONALITY

The clinical presentation of the dependent personality can be described in terms of behavioral and interpersonal styles, thinking style, and feeling style. The behavioral and interpersonal styles of people with this personality style are characterized by docility, passivity, and nonassertiveness. In interpersonal relations, they tend to be pleasing, self-sacrificing, clinging, and constantly requiring the assurance of others. Their compliance and reliance on others lead to a subtle demand that others assume responsibility for major areas of their lives.

The thinking or cognitive style of those with a dependent personality is characterized by suggestibility. They easily adopt a Pollyannaish attitude toward life. Furthermore, they tend to minimize difficulties, and because of this, their naiveté is easily persuadable and easily taken advantage of. In short, this style of thinking is uncritical and unperceptive.

Their feeling or affective style is characterized by insecurity and anxiousness. Because they lack self-confidence, they experience considerable discomfort at being alone. They tend to be preoccupied with the fear of abandonment and disapproval of others. Their mood tends to be one of anxiety or fearfulness, as well as having a somber or sad quality (Sperry, 2003a).

Development and Etiological Features

The following biopsychosocial formulation may be helpful in understanding how the dependent personality develops. Biologically, individuals with a dependent style are characterized by a low energy level. Their temperament is described as melancholic. As infants and young children, they were characterized as fearful, sad, or withdrawn. In terms of body types, they tend to have more endomorphic builds (Millon, 1981).

Psychologically, people with the dependent personality can be understood and appreciated in terms of their self-view, their worldview, and their life goal. The self-view of these individuals tends to be a variant of the theme "I'm nice, but inadequate [or fragile]." Their view of self is self-effacing, inept, and self-doubting. Their worldview is some variant of the theme "Others are here to take care of me, because I can't do it for myself." Their life goal is characterized by some variant of the theme "Therefore, cling to and rely on others at all cost."

The social features of this personality can be understood in terms of parental, familial, and environmental factors. The person with a dependent personality is most likely to have been raised in a family in which parental overprotection is prominent. It is as if the parental injunction to the child is "I can't trust you to do anything right [or well]." The person with a dependent style is likely to have been pampered and overprotected as a child. Contact with siblings and peers may engender feelings of unattractiveness, awkwardness, or competitive inadequacy, especially during the preadolescent and adolescent years. These can have a devastating impact on the individual and can further confirm the individual's sense of self-deprecation and doubt. The dependent personality becomes self-perpetuating through a process that involves a sense of self-doubt, an avoidance of competitive activity, and the availability of self-reliant individuals who are willing to take care of and make decisions for the person with a dependent style in exchange for his or her self-sacrificing and docile friendship (Sperry, 2003a).

Health-Related Dynamics

For clinicians, patients with a dependent personality provide a refreshing change of pace. These patients tend to be reliable, accommodating, and flattering until the real treatment needs to be done. At those times, they tend to be passive, and their lack of initiative may become a source of aggravation when they are faced with demands. Their coping style is characterized by displays of incompetency that effectively guarantee that caretaking will be available to them. When social support systems are lacking or inadequate, clinicians may need to find alternative sources of support, at least temporarily. Preventive health behaviors will occur only as long as these patients secure the attention and ongoing approval of strong, protective authority figures. Furthermore, diagnosis of their chronic disease will depend on the vigilance and acumen of the clinicians working with these patients. Once an illness is identified, they will conceptualize it in primitive terms, and it will provide them with various secondary gains, including achieving continual interpersonal contact with key relationships, getting others to make important decision for them, and neutralizing expressions of anger from frustrated clinicians and caretakers. Treatment adherence for such patients depends largely on the difficulty of the task and the extent of approval available if and when their effort is successful.

Although people with a dependent personality can be frustrating for clinicians to deal with during the course of their chronic illness, these patients will maintain their relationships with their clinicians and will be reasonably responsive, assuming that their limited capacity for independent functioning is not exceeded. Learning to become more self-reliant is essential. Success in achieving this goal requires considerable patience because the process tends to be slow and incremental. Though it requires ongoing encouragement and approval, the process also serves to strengthen the patient–clinician relationship.

Because of their childlike orientation, individuals with a dependent personality can be expected to rely on others to identify, as well as to solve, their health dilemmas because their ability to take charge of their lives can be quite limited. Another reason these patients are unlikely to direct much energy at health issues is that they are preoccupied with addressing interpersonal security needs during the course of their illness. Thus, they can appear to be oblivious to seemingly obvious disease-related emotional issues, such as postoperative pain or disability, which they assume their clinicians—whom they envision as omnipotent—will protect them from. When such eventualities do occur, their feelings of vulnerability and lack of personal control increase even further. They can become anxiety ridden because their expectation that others—including their clinicians—will care for them is shattered.

In acute medical situations in which a time-limited resolution is likely, improving the emotional course of their illness may involve coping by proxy, which effectively means that others, particularly their clinician, will do the work for them. However, when a chronic illness is involved, the situation is significantly more problematic. The clinician cannot assume that because he or she modeled useful coping behaviors for the patient, the intervention was somehow internalized. Instead, these individuals with a dependent style tend to regard the clinician as omnipotent and better suited to dealing with emotional issues than they are. Therefore, clinicians can provide gentle but firm insistence that the patient engage in specified tasks—for instance, make a phone call or write a letter—that begin to establish an interaction pattern that can be maintained for the duration of treatment. Assuming that the clinician closely monitors the patient and ensures that no substantial erosions occur with this plan and that judicious choices are made concerning what these patients can manage, the goal of increasing self-reliance can be incrementally achieved. In addition, the patients will experience increased self-confidence.

Illness detection and personal well-being for individuals with a dependent personality tends to be a secondary consideration for them, given their preoccupation with relationship security. To put it bluntly, self-preservation is relatively unimportant to them compared with securing and maintaining a relationship. Unless their illness is an important issue for a concerned partner, the patient with a dependent style can be expected to remain more focused on relationship preservation than on self-preservation.

The deferential, subordinating manner of those with a dependent personality has particularly important consequences for their illness management after the diagnosis of a chronic illness is made and treatment has begun. When authority figures recommend a particular course of action, the decision making of these patients may be determined more by the perceived stature of the recommending party than by a rational cost–benefit analysis. Their desire to please and accommodate their clinician may also lead these patients to distort or even misrepresent their illness status to ensure that their clinician will be satisfied. Unfortunately, the outcome of this attitude of relinquishment can be disastrous, particularly because, when symptoms are unreported, illness progression ensues. This may create disenchantment between clinician and patient, which can be quite threatening for either party.

Because of their poorly differentiated psychic organization, the manner in which patients with a dependent personality represent their illness can be childlike or primitive. Then, too, their impoverished sense of self can make it difficult for them to incorporate knowledge of their disease and disease management issues as personal knowledge. Instead, such information is more likely to be identified with their all-powerful clinician and embedded in the relationship rather than internalized by them. Although this appears to be a workable strategy when the clinician is available, attentive, and consistent, these conditions are less likely to exist in other treatment settings in which managed care or budget constraints limit patient–clinician contacts or when continuity of care is fragmented.

When their disease is likely to distress or negatively affect their primary relationship, as for instance, breast cancer may do, an element of desperation is added. Accordingly, the clinician will have to remain alert to the meaning and significance of this relationship to their patients, particularly those with dependent personality disorder, so that specific interventions, such as couple counseling, can be provided in times of need. It is not surprising that anxiety and depression are likely consequences and that at times such patients may require pharmacological support in addition to focused psychotherapy (Harper, 2003).

The Experience of Diabetes

Because diabetes represents an ongoing demand for self-management, this chronic illness is a particularly difficult condition for patients with a dependent personality. Given the limited incentive to engage in disciplined behavior by patients with a dependent personality, the clinicians' expectations for them to engage in daily self-monitoring, self-denial, and self-regulation are likely to be ignored. Thus, from the onset of the diagnosis of diabetes, it is important that the notion of self-discipline as an essential element of illness management be discussed with these patients. It is also essential to elicit whatever apprehensions and concerns this idea may engender in them.

Demands and expectations placed on the patient with a dependent style need to be manageable and achievable so that success is relatively assured both in the beginning and in the later stages of treatment. When difficulties arise, it is better to view these difficulties as opportunities for conjoint problem solving rather than as failures. This reframing can enhance the sense of closeness needed for a long-term medical relationship. In a way, this strategy represents a reversal of what typically takes place in medical practice, wherein the absence of a symptom or health problem results in a reduction of contact, that is, appointments, with the nurturing authority figure. For individuals with a dependent personality, who are continually seeking security and caretaking, such an attitude constitutes a negative model for illness management. Accordingly, ample opportunities for these patients to report success and effective regulation of blood sugar levels are needed, especially in the early stages of promoting this important health behavior. This means that a fixed, ongoing schedule of appointments is recommended.

Treating diabetes in patients with a dependent personality is best conceptualized as a shared concern and conjoint undertaking that reinforces the need by these patients to feel a part of the treatment process, a secure and attention-providing atmosphere. Emphasizing periodic follow-ups wherein enthusiastic recognition is provided for their health maintenance efforts in the face of a potentially serious disease can help reinforce these patients' positive attitude toward maintaining a disciplined approach to illness management. It is also useful in engendering an increased sense of self-efficacy wherein their security needs are assured and even enhanced by their active participation in the treatment process (Harper, 2003).

AVOIDANT PERSONALITY

People with an avoidant personality are seemingly shy, lonely, hypersensitive individuals with low self-esteem. Although they are desperate for interpersonal involvement, they avoid personal contact with others because of their heightened fear of social disapproval and their rejection sensitivity. In this regard, they are quite different from the schizoid personality, who has little, if any, interest in personal contact. The avoidant personality style is characterized by the following behavioral and interpersonal styles, thinking or cognitive style, and emotional or affective style. The behavioral style of those with an avoidant personality is characterized by social withdrawal, shyness, distrustfulness, and aloofness. Their behavior and speech are both controlled and inactive, and they appear apprehensive and awkward. Interpersonally, they are rejection sensitive. Even though they desire acceptance by others, they keep their distance from others and require unconditional approval before being willing to "open up." They gradually "test" others to determine who can be trusted to like them (Sperry, 2003a).

Development and Etiological Features

The following biopsychosocial formulation may be helpful in understanding how the avoidant personality style is likely to have developed. Biologically, individuals with an avoidant style exhibit a low energy level. Their temperament is usually of the melancholic type, and as infants and young children, they were characterized as sad, fearful, and withdrawn (Millon, 1981).

Psychologically, these individuals can be understood and appreciated by their characteristic self-view, worldview, and life goal. They tend to see the world as some variant of the theme "Life is unfair—people reject and criticize me—but I still want someone to like me." As such, they are likely to conclude, "Therefore, be vigilant, demand reassurance, and if all else fails, fantasize and daydream about the way life could be." The most common defense mechanism of someone with an avoidant personality is that of fantasy.

Socially, predictable patterns of parenting and environmental factors can be noted for the avoidant personality disorder. The person with an avoidant personality is likely to have experienced parental rejection and ridicule. Later, siblings and peers will likely continue this pattern of rejection and ridicule. The parental injunction is likely to have been "We don't accept you, and probably no one else will either." They may have had parents with high standards, and they worried that they may not have met or would not meet these standards and therefore would not be accepted.

This avoidant pattern is confirmed, reinforced, and perpetuated by the following individual and systems factors: A sense of personal inadequacy and a fear of rejection lead to hypervigilance, which leads to restricted social experiences. These experiences, plus catastrophic thinking, lead to increased hypervigilance and hypersensitivity, leading to self-pity, anxiety, and depression, which lead to further confirmation of avoidant beliefs and styles (Sperry, 2003a).

Health-Related Dynamics

Ideally, patients with an avoidant personality approach health care with the best of intentions; however, the reality is that their primary goal is to avoid the censure and disapproval of those with whom they are dealing. During routine, uncomplicated medical encounters such as annual checkups, health care providers tend to be quite pleased, and these patients will be reasonably comfortable. However, when interactions and the treatment regimen are complex or aversive, such as when a physician is brusque, then the patient's characteristic apprehensiveness and rejection sensitivity will emerge as a complicating factor. Because of their avoidant coping strategy, they are less likely than other patients to engage in efforts to seek needed social support, to clarify needed medical information, and to effectively monitor and report on their symptoms. In situations in which they anticipate censure, criticism, or rejection, individuals who are avoidant are likely to retreat into a private, anxious world cut off from corrective opportunities and to ruminate on thoughts of worthlessness and self-loathing. It is not surprising that they reflectively pull back from opportunities that might offer needed social support for themselves. Unless their symptoms are severe enough to overcome their typical avoidance pattern, help seeking is delayed or reduced, which lessens the probability of early disease detection. The way in which they represent illness to themselves and others tends to be infused with anxious preoccupation and heightened fears of nonacceptance. Therefore, it is also not surprising that these attitudes and behaviors are not conducive to an accurate understanding of their disease process and its management. Underuse of health care resources is more likely, given that these individuals predictably shy away from unfamiliar social contacts, especially those involving group formats. Secondary gain will center on relief from anxiety, stemming from aversive social contact or performance situations in which failure or criticism is possible.

Clinicians endeavoring to work effectively with individuals with an avoidant personality need to adopt a patient, accepting, and nurturing orientation in their initial meeting with these patients. Recognizing that these patients are all too often "lost to follow-up," clinicians need to anticipate their fear and reluctance and plan and implement strategies that ensure that ongoing contact is maintained. Given the tendency of people with an avoidant personality toward social isolation and their anxious, ruminative style, clinicians must expect these patients to be initially difficult to engage in the treatment process but that an intentional strategy of patience, understanding, and nurturance will, in time, be rewarded with appreciation and commitment to the treatment team and the treatment process.

The initial impression of these patients is that they are quiet, passively compliant individuals who are socially responsive but who maintain a distance that makes establishing a comfortable patient–clinician relationship in the first few sessions unlikely. However, they are not difficult patients to work with, particularly if there are no complicated medical conditions or procedures involved. But when medical conditions require extended interactions, particularly those involving emotional exchanges, problems can emerge that may be perplexing to the clinician. At such times, the characteristic defensive maneuvers of the avoidant personality style are activated. In their efforts to avoid ridicule or rejection, and to keep from being viewed as stupid, patients who are avoidant may passively acknowledge their understanding of medical treatment regimens even when they do not really understand them. When clinicians communicate their frustration with, or disapproval of, the patients' nonadherence to treatment, these patients will feel rejected and, not unexpectedly, may abandon treatment entirely or seek out another health care provider to escape additional rejection.

Similarly, in order not be viewed as a bother, these patients may fail to report important complaint information necessary for symptom monitoring or effective medical management. Unless the clinician recognizes that such nonadherence is an inadvertent feature of the avoidant personality style, the irritation that this engenders in the clinician is likely to be perceived by the patient as confirmation that the clinician does not really care about him or her and is just as critical and rejecting as everyone else in the patient's life. Needless to say, the kind of supportive, caring, tolerant, and patient orientation that these patients require may be beyond the capacity of many busy physicians. Thus, it is essential that someone in that practice—a nurse or other health care professional—invest the time, caring, and interest in such patients.

The social skill deficits of individuals with an avoidant personality become accentuated in the course of their illness, because the treatment process necessarily places them in a dependent stance with strangers, on whose goodwill their lives depends. Illness also tends to displace these individuals from their carefully contrived, insular social environment and typically thrusts them into a busy and often impersonal health care setting, which is more than most individuals can manage, particularly when a debilitating, chronic disease is involved. For the patient with an avoidant personality whose social fears exceed those of all other patients, it means that they must cope with an additional and significant array of troubling stressors, above and beyond those of the disease itself.

Because the anguish of patients with an avoidant style is generally internalized, their external behavior appears confusing and frustrating to health care personnel. What is observed is a haphazard, fragmented response to medical treatment demands and erratic treatment adherence efforts, which are common markers of the so-called difficult patient. It is not surprising that health care providers do not particularly like such patients and so they attempt to confront, avoid, or limit their contact with them, which only serves to reinforce the individual's isolation and feelings of rejection and self-loathing. Rather than a using a confrontational approach with individuals who are avoidant, a supportive, empathic orientation that recognizes the difficulties that these individuals face will help them focus on the threats they must address. Otherwise, those with an avoidant personality disorder may engage in purposefully disruptive activities that momentarily protect them from perceived threats but also prevent effective problem resolution. When important medical decision making must be accomplished rapidly, people with an avoidant style may lack the assertive skills to ask appropriate questions or to articulate their personal doubts or concerns when confronted with an impatient medical practitioner.

In such conflictual interpersonal circumstances, clinicians sensitive to behavioral medicine issues can be quite helpful. Such a clinician can consult with members of the patient's health care team and clarify how the patient's intrapersonal dynamics impact interpersonal processes. The clinician can suggest interpersonal strategies for gaining patient confidence and facilitate relationship building. Furthermore, the clinician can consult with such patients by helping them construct a hierarchy of concerns, questions, and adherence requirements related to their illness management. These patients can also be assisted in dealing with the specific interpersonal encounters (Harper, 2003).

The Experience of Diabetes

Because individuals with an avoidant personality are anxiety prone, stressful situations can significantly alter their glucose metabolism. Dealing with such glucose fluctuations that are not diet related can be a source of interpersonal tension and recrimination with the health care providers, who are unlikely to consider alternative causes and instead attribute difficulty to patient misbehavior or nonadherence. Such a misunderstanding can result in a sense of rejection potentially strong enough that troubled patients who are avoidant might exit the health care system entirely. Once rejected, these patients may remain fearful about seeking alternative care, which they would anticipate as ultimately rejecting. Therefore, health care providers need to manifest patience and a patient-centered orientation in relating to such patients, as well as engage in discussion and monitoring of all stressful factors that contribute to problematic blood sugar regulation (Harper, 2003).

NARCISSISTIC PERSONALITY

The narcissistic personality is characterized by the following behavioral and interpersonal styles, cognitive style, and affective style. Behaviorally, individuals with a narcissistic personality are seen as conceited, boastful, and snobbish. They appear self-assured and self-centered, and they tend to dominate conversation, seek admiration, and act in a pompous and exhibitionistic fashion. They are also impatient, arrogant, and thin skinned or hypersensitive. Interpersonally, they are exploitive and use others to indulge themselves and their desires. Their behavior is socially facile, pleasant, and endearing. However, they are unable to respond with true empathy toward others. When stressed, they can be disdainful, exploitive, and generally irresponsible in their behavior.

Their thinking style is one of cognitive expansiveness and exaggeration. They tend to focus on images and themes rather than on facts and issues. In fact, they take liberties with the facts, distort them, and even engage in prevarication and self-deception to preserve their own illusions about themselves and the projects in which they are involved. Their cognitive style is also marked by inflexibility. In addition, they have an exaggerated sense of self-importance and establish unrealistic goals of power, wealth, and ability. They justify all of this with their sense of entitlement and exaggerated sense of their own self-importance.

Their feeling or affective style is characterized by an aura of self-confidence and nonchalance, which is present in most situations except when their narcissistic confidence is shaken. Then they are likely to respond with rage at criticism. Their feelings toward others shift and vacillate between overidealization and devaluation. Finally, their inability to show empathy is reflected in their superficial relationships with minimal emotional ties or commitments (Sperry, 2003a).

Developmental and Etiological Features

The following biopsychosocial formulation may be helpful in understanding how the narcissistic personality disorder is likely to have developed. Biologically, people with a narcissistic personality tend to have hyperresponsive temperaments (Millon, 1981). As young children, they were viewed by others as being special in terms of looks, talents, or "promise." Often as young children, they had early and exceptional speech development. In addition, they were likely keenly aware of interpersonal cues.

Psychologically, people with narcissism view themselves, others, the world, and life's purpose in terms of the following themes: "I'm special and unique, and I am entitled to extraordinary rights and privileges whether I have earned them or not." Their worldview is a variant of the theme "Life is a banquet table to be sampled at will. People owe me admiration and privilege." Their goal is "Therefore, I'll expect and demand this specialness." Common defense mechanisms used by the person with a narcissistic personality involve rationalization and projective identification.

Socially, predictable parental patterns and environmental factors can be noted for people with the narcissistic style. Parental indulgence and overevaluation characterize their narcissistic personality. The parental injunction was likely "Grow up and be wonderful—for me." Often they were only children and, in addition, may have sustained early losses in childhood. From an early age, they learned exploitive and manipulative behavior from their parents. This narcissistic pattern is confirmed, reinforced, and perpetuated by certain individual and systems factors. The illusion of specialness, disdain for others' views, and a sense of entitlement lead to an underdeveloped sense of social interest and responsibility. This, in turn, leads to increased self-absorption and confirmation of narcissistic beliefs (Sperry, 2003a).

Health-Related Dynamics

When physically healthy, individuals who are narcissistic can come across as superficially gracious and charming, with a sense of importance and invulnerability. However, when confronted with chronic illness and thrust into the subservient role of patient, these individuals come across entirely differently. Their need to be superior will drive them to undermine medical authority roles and cast health care personnel into the role of servants. It is not surprising that this generates considerable resentment and conflict and can seriously undermine the treatment process. They tend to be exploitive of social supports and engage in entitled, demanding behavior. Requests that they engage in preventive measures is typically dismissed as beneath them. Consequently, diagnosis of their chronic disease may be delayed by their overconfidence in their health status and may result in disbelief or, conversely, panic and deflation if their perceived sense of superiority is threatened. Their inflated but fragile self-esteem undoubtedly contributes to distortions in the manner in which they represent and conceptualize their illness to themselves and others. Treatment adherences issues are complicated by the tendency of the patient with narcissism to devalue and reject demeaning self-management recommendations. Their behavior may be especially abusive when they feel most threatened and vulnerable. Overall, a clinical strategy of managing these patients with a combination of respect and authority often determines the success and effectiveness of their treatment.

Typically, patients with a narcissistic personality present an interpersonal challenge to physicians, given that their often presumptuous and arrogant manner is offensive to most physicians, particularly those who view themselves as experts or authority figures. Needless to say, when a chronic illness is involved, the likelihood of these patient's disruptive confrontation and alienation increases. Unfortunately, that animosity created by such interpersonal behavior can greatly complicate treatment and the use of health care resources, sometimes even inadvertently affecting the very health of these patients.

Curiously, physical illness can have a diminishing effect on the grandiose aspirations and expectations of the patient with a narcissistic style. To the degree that a threatening diagnosis represents an assault on this patient's sense of omnipotence, the health care provider may too easily be perceived as the bearer of bad tidings and subsequently become the target of punishment and retribution. For patients with narcissism, the prospect of taking on the patient role, which implies vulnerability and dependence on others, is totally unacceptable, so they may attempt to recast their relationship with health care providers by treating them as servants whose duty it is to restore their health.

There is considerable variability among those with a narcissistic personality in coping with their illness. When bravado and optimism can be adaptive, such individuals may manifest an adequate capacity to cope with emotional issues, and their ability to enlist others to ensure their needs get met can result in effective problem-solving behavior, at least initially. However, difficulties are likely to emerge when the demands of emotional and problem-solving coping become simultaneously confounded with one another. Then, interpersonally abrasive problem solving can precipitate an interpersonal crisis requiring emotion-focused coping that competes with emotional issues pertaining to their disease. The result may be that necessary planning or completion of specific responsibilities is delayed or derailed.

Chronic illness forces these individuals into a dependent role requiring reliance on the goodwill of others. Before their diagnosis, some patients who are narcissistic could use looks, power, wealth, resources, or talents to seduce, coerce, or intimidate others into doing what they wanted, whereas other such patients who are unattractive or have limited financial means were unlikely to succeed by acting in such a fashion. However, when chronically ill, these narcissistic individuals can likewise be demanding and arrogant. Remarkably, their forceful manner and sense of conviction that they are justified in their demands can intimidate physicians into making medical decisions that previously might not be considered. Arguably, the inflammatory and antagonistic nature of their behavior can result in either patients or physicians "firing" the other, with the subsequent disruption of efficient health care use. Although physicians sometimes become the targets of these patients' rage, it is more likely that subordinates will take the brunt of it. Because these patients can defer the authority of the physician, initially the physician may not understand the resentment and antagonism experienced by the rest of the treatment team.

As health care professionals become able to recognize the inherent vulnerability of patients with a narcissistic personality, these professionals are more able to tolerate their abrasive style. After being humiliated by confrontation with greater authority, such patients may feel impelled to seek vindictive retribution. Therefore, maintaining a state of respectful formality, firm politeness, and professionalism rather than openly confronting these patients is the preferred way of interacting with them. This strategy offers a realistic and effective means of maintaining a needed sense of control in the relationship. Furthermore, ignoring minor slights and overfamiliarities while expressing one's authority implicitly through displays of professional knowledge allows the health care provider to maintain a task-oriented climate in the relationship. Similarly, the patient's unreasonable and excessive requests or demands can be politely declined with appropriate justifications or deferred for later consideration.

Finally, clinicians who consult with health providers facing the inevitable aversive encounters associated with patients with narcissistic personality disorder do well to encourage and foster debriefing. More specifically, debriefing is introduced and demonstrated for staff—particularly support staff, who are the usual targets of the snide remarks, demands, and ragefulness of the patient with narcissism. Debriefing is helpful in ventilating frustrations, in regaining perspective, and in maintaining the professional focus necessary for high-quality health care.

Staff can increase these patients' investment in their treatment by providing them formal briefings regarding their health status, their treatment plan, and, when appropriate, the opportunity to participate in decision making. Scheduling meeting times convenient to the staff, rather than to the patient, can maintain an atmosphere of formality as well as regulated, respectful interactions (Harper, 2003).

The Experience of Diabetes

Diabetes requires ongoing vigilance, self-monitoring, and a willingness to engage in self-denial of foods and other activities that can adversely affect blood sugar levels. Individuals preoccupied with lofty fantasies of their own self-importance are not well suited to the humbling task of self-discipline that diabetes requires. The presence of a spouse who is responsible for meal preparation can be invaluable in establishing and maintaining limits to the patient's tendency toward self-indulgent excesses. However, the spouse may also bear the brunt of his or her partner's frustration in the form of displaced anger over such constraints. Cavalier and dismissive behavior should be expected from patients with a narcissistic style, who may perceive and treat their condition as the medical team's responsibility. Even if these patients pay limited lip service to health care directives, even small deviations from full compliance can have long-range health consequences.

An overall strategy for working with these patients is to emphasize simple, straightforward, and easy-to-use directives. This contrasts with the typical medical care counseling directive, which emphasizes the importance of long-range adherence and the future risk of complications if ignored. Such directives tend to have little impact on people with a narcissistic personality because of the absence of dramatic immediate consequences, for instance, of continuing to smoke. Such patients tend to react in a condescending manner to physicians and other health personnel who might recommend something like smoking cessation. Their condescending and provocative behavior in the face of medical knowledge about their condition and long-range risk can be infuriating and can test the resolve of many physicians who might be tempted to "fire" such individuals from their practice. The more burdensome the routines required to control diabetes, the more unlikely these patients will be to make and keep such a commitment. However, devices such as insulin pumps that require minimal patient involvement represent a highly cost-effective investment. Maintaining sufficient rapport so that the patient keeps appointments is essential to ensure early identification and treatment of complications associated with progression of the debilitating disease, such as retinal changes, peripheral neuropathy, or renal changes and dysfunction (Harper, 2003).

BORDERLINE PERSONALITY

The borderline personality is characterized by the following behavior and interpersonal styles, cognitive style, and emotional style. Behaviorally, people with a borderline personality are characterized by physically self-damaging acts such as suicide gestures, self-mutilation, or the provocation of fights. Their social and occupational accomplishments are often less than their intelligence and ability warrant. Of all the personality disorders, they are more likely to have irregularities of circadian rhythms, especially of the sleep–wake cycle. Thus, chronic insomnia is a common complaint. Interpersonally, people with a borderline style are characterized by their paradoxical instability. That is, they fluctuate quickly between idealizing and clinging to another individual to devaluing and opposing that individual. They are exquisitely rejection sensitive, and experience abandonment depression following the slightest of stressors. Millon (1981) considered separation anxiety as a primary motivator of this personality disorder. Interpersonal relationships develop rather quickly and intensely, yet their social adaptiveness is rather superficial. They are extraordinarily intolerant of being alone, and they go to great lengths to seek out the company of others, whether in indiscriminate sexual affairs, late-night phone calls to relatives and recent acquaintances, or late-night visits to hospital emergency rooms with a host of vague medical or psychiatric complaints.

Their cognitive style is described as inflexible and impulsive (Millon, 1981). Inflexibility of their style is characterized by rigid abstractions that easily lead to grandiose, idealized perceptions of others, not as real people, but as personifications of "all good" or "all bad" individuals. They reason by analogy from past experience and thus have difficulty reasoning logically and learning from past experiences and relationships. Because they have an external locus of control, people with a borderline personality usually blame others when things go wrong. By accepting responsibility for their own incompetence, those who have a borderline style believe they would feel even more powerless to change their circumstances. Accordingly, their emotions fluctuate between hope and despair because they believe that external circumstances are well beyond their control. Their cognitive style is also marked by impulsivity, and just as they vacillate between idealization and devaluation of others, their thoughts shift from one extreme to another: "I like people, no I don't like them"; "Having goals is good, no it's not"; "I need to get my life together, no I can't, it's hopeless." This inflexibility and impulsivity complicate the process of identity formation. Their uncertainty about self-image, gender identity, goals, values, and career choice reflects their impulsive and inflexible stance. Their inflexibility and impulsivity are further noted in their tendency toward "splitting." *Splitting* is the inability to synthesize contradictory qualities, such that the individual views others as all good or all bad and uses projective identification, that is, attributing one's own negative or dangerous feelings to others. Their cognitive style is further characterized by an inability to tolerate frustration. Finally, micropsychotic episodes can be noted when these individuals are under a great deal of stress. These are ill-defined, strange thought processes especially noted in response to unstructured rather than structured situations and may take the form of derealization, depersonalization, intense rage reactions, unusual reactions to drugs, and intense brief paranoid episodes. Because of difficulty in focusing attention and subsequent loss of relevant data, people with a borderline personality also have a diminished capacity to process information.

The emotional style of individuals with this disorder is characterized by marked mood shifts from a normal or euthymic mood to a dysphoric mood. In addition, inappropriate and intense anger and rage may easily be triggered. On the other extreme are feelings of emptiness, a deep "void," or boredom (Sperry, 2003a).

Developmental and Etiological Features

The following biopsychosocial formulation may be helpful in understanding how the borderline personality pattern is likely to have developed. Biologically, people with a borderline personality can be understood in terms of the three main subtypes: borderline–dependent, borderline–histrionic, and borderline–passive–aggressive. The temperamental style of a person with the borderline–dependent subtype is that of the passive infantile pattern (Millon, 1981). Millon (1981) hypothesized that low autonomic nervous system reactivity plus an overprotective parenting style facilitates restrictive interpersonal skills and a clinging relational style. However, a person with the histrionic subtype was more likely to have a hyperresponsive infantile pattern. Thus, because of high autonomic nervous system reactivity and increased parental stimulation and expectations for performance, the borderline–histrionic pattern is likely to result. Finally, the temperamental style of a person who is borderline–passive–aggressive was likely to have been the "difficult child" type noted by Thomas and Chess (1977). This pattern, plus parental inconsistency, marks the affective irritability of someone with a borderline–passive–aggressive personality.

Psychologically, people with a borderline personality tend to view themselves, others, the world, and life's purpose in terms of the following themes. They view themselves by some variant of the theme "I don't know who I am or where I'm going." In short, their identity problems involve gender, career, loyalties, and values, and their self-esteem fluctuates with each thought or feeling about their self-identity. They also tend to view their world with some variant of the theme "People are great, no they are not"; "Having goals is good, no it's not"; or "If life doesn't go my way, I can't tolerate it." Accordingly, they are likely to conclude, "Therefore, keep all options open. Don't commit to anything. Reverse roles and vacillate thinking and feelings when under attack." The most common defense mechanisms used by individuals with a borderline personality disorder are regression, splitting, and projective identification.

Socially, predictable patterns of parenting and environmental factors can be noted for the borderline personality disorder. Parenting style differs depending on the subtype. For example, in patients with the dependent subtype, overprotectiveness characterizes parenting, whereas in those with the histrionic subtype, a demanding parenting style is more evident, and an inconsistent parenting style is more noted in patients with the passive–aggressive subtype. But because the borderline personality disorder is a syndromal elaboration and deterioration of the less severe dependent, histrionic, or passive–aggressive personality disorders, the family of origin in those with the borderline subtype of these disorders is likely to be much more dysfunctional, increasing the likelihood that the child will have learned various self-defeating coping strategies. The parental injunction is likely to have been "If you grow up and leave me, bad things will happen to me [parent]."

This borderline pattern is confirmed, reinforced, and perpetuated by the following individual and systems factors: Diffuse identity, impulsive vacillation, and self-defeating coping strategies lead to aggressive acting out, which leads to more chaos, which leads to the experience of depersonalization, increased dysphoria, or self-mutilation to achieve some relief. This leads to further reconfirmation of their beliefs about self and the world, as well as reinforcement of the behavioral and interpersonal patterns (Sperry, 2003a).

Health-Related Dynamics

Individuals with a borderline personality are characterized by lability and instability, which is evident, in one form or other, in all medical encounters. Even when only a mild disease process is present, the clinician may still observe their behavioral excesses in the form of substance abuse, self-destructive behavior, and disorganized symptom presentations related to episodic decompensation. However, it is during the course of chronic illness that the pathology of the borderline personality pattern is most evident. Initially, the social behavior of these individuals can be engaging or charming, but as relationships become more intense and complicated, that treatment becomes confounded or diverted by the their tendency to fragment relationships, to display splitting and help-seeking behaviors, and to alternate displays of dependency and rage. Their acute sensitivity to the vulnerabilities of others, including physicians and nurses, inevitably seems to draws them into conflict. Preventive health behavior efforts tend to be inconsistent and haphazard, ranging from the extremes of overidentification with the pursuit of wellness to total disregard of health concern or self-destructive indulgence. Because they are consumed with relational issues and personal identity conflicts, disease detection is an afterthought for them. Then, when a chronic disease is diagnosed, even if their illness representation is accurate, it tends to be highly emotionally charged and liable to distortion by subsequent relational changes. Adhering to treatment regimens is predictably erratic for these patients and is often characterized by nonadherence as they act out in protest any relational conflicts or dissatisfactions.

Similarly, their under- and overuse of health care resources is predicated on the current status of their relationships. Secondary gain is not uncommon and typically takes several forms. These include escape from conflicts regarding intimacy and trust, the use of illness to escape retribution, and a perverse satisfaction in triggering anger in health care providers frustrated by their irresponsible behavior. Depending on the severity of their psychopathology and lability of affect and mood should dictate whether a nonpsychologically trained clinician should engage these patients in transference issues when they arise, or whether expert consultation from a psychotherapist who is experienced with borderline pathology in medical settings is indicated. Even if these patients are undergoing psychotherapy, it may well be that the course of medical treatment will still be discomforting to all involved.

Patients with a borderline personality typically possess adequate social skills and demeanor when they are in nondistressing circumstances. However, distress, particularly relational stress, negatively impacts them, as witnessed by their inability to tolerate frustrations, sustain relationships, and maintain a coherent, consistent course of action. Moving from relationship to relationship characterizes people with a borderline personality style. To the extent to which they are sufficiently attractive and personable, they may be able to forestall serious, debilitating decompensation by moving on to a new relationship. But it is when they are constrained in a relationship, by external circumstances or by their own psychological dependency, that their own vulnerabilities emerge in crisis proportions. It is not surprising that a serious, chronic illness may provoke such a crisis by constraining patients with a borderline style in several ways. Because a chronic illness tends to increase their dependence on others, they cling to others even more so to meet their basic needs, such as money if they are unable to work, transportation if they cannot drive, and shopping if they are bedridden, as well as other disease-specific activities. These are examples of problem-focused coping that is disrupted by illness episodes that keep them from performing those activities themselves. All these demands and consequences accumulate, increasing their stress burden, in addition to reducing their level of energy and the negative feelings associated with a chronic illness.

Any individual with a chronic illness finds him- or herself relying increasingly on significant others, family members, medical personnel, and various agencies for assistance. Social convention requires some minimal reciprocity in the form of at least superficial cordiality and appreciation of helpers. This demand can be particularly problematic for patients with a borderline personality, given their erratic, capricious style of interpersonal relating. It should not be too surprising that often helpers cower at the thought of having to deal with such patients.

Emotionally focused coping is another significant issue for these individuals. They are poorly equipped to cope emotionally, given their chronic mood instability and the reverberations of their erratic interpersonal behaviors. In addition to dealing poorly with emotional- and problem-focused aspects of the chronic illness confronting them, these patients' chaotic interpersonal conduct often alienates others, further heightening their sense of instability and insecurity. It also undermines their efforts to manage their illness or recovery.

Unfortunately, their chronic disease can become a secondary issue to the emotional crisis that can itself threaten treatment or recovery. Early detection of their instabilities and the involvement of clinicians experienced in dealing with the complicated management issues their treatment poses can minimize much suffering for these patients. It can also decrease health care expenses in terms of both dollar cost and the distress incurred by the health care providers involved with this individual's treatment (Harper, 2003).

The Experience of Diabetes

Like others with chronic illnesses that require self-monitoring, self-discipline, and consistency, patients with a borderline personality, as well as their health providers, face a constant challenge in dealing with diabetes. Lability and overmodulated affect are reflected in endocrine surges; thus, maintaining stable blood sugar levels is a major challenge for these patients. This instability is complicated by impulsive dietary indiscretion, substance abuse, and nicotine and caffeine use—which greatly constricts small blood vessels—as well as inattention to or neglect of insulin regulation because of emotional interpersonal conflicts. Being accountable for such health behaviors—for instance, maintaining stable blood sugar levels—requires psychological requisites lacking in most patients with a borderline style. These include a cohesive sense of self and the capacity to modulate affect. Even in psychologically mature people with diabetes, maintaining a resolve to resist temptation is a difficult and significant accomplishment, often taken for granted by physicians and other health care providers.

Even though patients with a borderline personality disorder may intellectually accept the responsibility to be accountable for maintaining stable blood sugar levels to prevent long-range complications, emotionally they find actualizing this promise extraordinarily difficult. Usually, the planning phase for chronic illness management is not necessarily problematic for these patients, unless they are smokers or obesity is a primary contributor to their illness. It is the action or implementation phase of the treatment plan that is predictability problematic. Even if they are initially successful in implementing a diet and blood sugar monitoring plan, maintaining it without relapse or departing from the schedule tends to be their downfall. Although adverse physical consequences of poor control may have a transient sobering effect on these individuals at the time the indiscretions occur, these are not likely to serve as effective determinants of future health-related behaviors. Because such patients' lability and instability are usually triggered by interpersonal issues, monitoring the relational aspect of their lives clearly must become an essential component of their treatment management. Self-neglect during a relationship conflict can precipitate a diabetic crisis, such as a coma. This usually occurs because the patient transiently decompensates and forgets to take insulin or deliberately stops taking insulin to elicit guilt or remorse from his or her partner or family. Similarly, if such patients binge eat or drink excessively, their blood sugar levels can become unstable and result in a crisis. Knowing that these scenarios are possible and predicting the likelihood that they will occur should prompt an action plan. For example, if the relationships of patients with diabetes are typically tumultuous and fragile, psychotherapy probably should be regarded as an essential component of their medical management (Harper, 2003).

CONCLUDING NOTE

This chapter has sketched portraits of six personality types, that is, styles or disorders, commonly encountered in health care contexts. The unique personality dynamics of each of these types were described with an emphasis on health-related dynamics, particularly illness representations and characteristic responses to clinicians and the treatment process. For any reader who might have doubted that chronic illness is experienced differently by patients, the vastly differing portrayals of the experience of diabetes challenges that assumption. These portrayals also suggest that clinicians who can recognize and understand these styles and can tailor their practice style accordingly are likely to be more effective and confident in patient encounters.

II

THE BIOPSYCHOSOCIAL THERAPY APPROACH TO CHRONIC ILLNESS

5

THE BIOPSYCHOSOCIAL THERAPY APPROACH TO CHRONIC ILLNESS: AN OVERVIEW

Biopsychosocial Therapy is an integrative approach for conceptualizing and implementing treatment when biological factors present along with psychological and sociocultural factors. Based on the biopsychosocial model (Engel, 1977), it is an integrative approach in two ways. First, it integrates or strategically combines various treatment modalities—individual, group, couple or family counseling, and medication—as well as various methods—dynamic, cognitive–behavioral, systemic, and psychoeducational. Second, it integrates and tailors these modalities and methods to the needs, styles, and expectations of the patient, be it an individual patient, a couple, or a family.

By definition, chronic medical illnesses have a biological substrate or base on which they influence and are influenced by psychological and sociocultural dynamics. Because of the presence of this biological base, clinicians—whether they are medical or nonmedical therapists—must formulate or conceptualize cases in biological as well as psychosocial terms. Such biopsychosocial formulations usually lead to treatment plans that combine biological modalities with psychosocial ones. Although biological modalities usually refer to medication, they also include nutrition modification, exercise prescription, and alternative remedies such as nutriceuticals (e.g., vitamins and herbal preparations). Although using certain biological modalities in psychotherapy may be outside the clinician's scope of practice, effective, ethical treatment requires appropriate referral and collaboration. For this and other reasons noted in the book, Biopsychosocial Therapy can be valuable to psychotherapists and other clinicians working with individuals with chronic illness.

This chapter begins by describing the history and development of the Biopsychosocial Therapy approach. It then explains some of the basic premises underlying this approach. Next, it overviews the four phases of Biopsychosocial Therapy and presents common clinical indications for this approach. It also interrelates the phase model of illness with the four phases of treatment of the Biopsychosocial Therapy approach. Finally, treatment goals are addressed. The last section discusses common goals in treating patients with chronic illness—both process goals and outcome goals.

HISTORY AND DEVELOPMENT OF
BIOPSYCHOSOCIAL THERAPY

Biopsychosocial Therapy is a systematically eclectic approach to therapeutic intervention that I formally described and first articulated in 1988 (Sperry, 1988, 1999a, 2000, 2001a, 200lb). Rather than referring to it as a uniquely new treatment approach, I prefer to think of it as an articulation and systemization of a way of conceptualizing treatment planning based on biopsychosocial and teleological principles. Because of its comprehensive and integrative emphasis, it is particularly appropriate for cases that are termed *difficult* or *treatment resistant* or when there is comorbidity of various medical and psychiatric conditions. This, of course, includes chronic physical illness.

Prior to my clinical experience as an attending physician and professor in the departments of psychiatry and behavioral medicine, family medicine, and preventive medicine at a major medical school and academic medical center, I successfully practiced a single-modality–oriented psychotherapy with relatively high-functioning individuals in a private practice setting. Unfortunately, the success I experienced with this approach did not translate well to the difficult-to-treat individuals who were routinely referred to our tertiary care treatment clinic by frustrated single-modality–oriented clinicians in the community. Most of these difficult-to-treat individuals had one or more chronic diseases.

It did not take long before I became acquainted with and embraced the biopsychosocial model. As described by Engel (1977), the biopsychosocial model is a holistic perspective for understanding and explaining the interfacing biological, psychological, and social forces that influence health, illness, and well-being. More specifically, an adequate understanding and explanation of an individual's situation is possible only when the clinician considers the biological, psychological, and social dimensions impacting the individual, because a holistic and multidimensional explanation is more powerful and complete than simply a psychological, biological, or social explanation. The obvious corollary was that a biopsychosocial and multidimensional understanding should be followed by biopsychosocial, multidimensional, and multimodal treatment interventions. Thereafter, I evaluated all patients from a biopsychosocial perspective. While I continued to use a single-modality approach with psychotherapy patients whose issues were primarily psychological, I sought to plan and implement multidimensional, multimodal interventions with those patients whose issues were broader. I came to call this approach *Biopsychosocial Therapy* (Sperry, 1988, 1999a, 2000, 2001a, 2001b). In short, Biopsychosocial Therapy is an integrative and systematic strategy for conceptualizing and implementing treatment based on biopsychosocial principles.

BASIC PREMISES OF BIOPSYCHOSOCIAL THERAPY

The four basic theoretical assumptions or premises that underlie Biopsychosocial Therapy are briefly noted and described in the following list:

1. *Biopsychosocial model.* As noted in chapter 3, the biopsychosocial model is a holistic perspective for understanding and explaining the interfacing biological, psychological, and social forces that influence health, illness, and well-being. Biopsychosocial Therapy is the articulation of that model for the clinical practice of psychotherapy and other psychologically informed treatment approaches.

2. *Wellness and integration as outcomes.* In chapter 1, *health status* was distinguished from *wellness*. Three distinct ranges of health status and wellness can be specified: the disordered range, the adequate range, and the optimal range. The goal of much therapy—particularly when reimbursed by third-party payers—is to move patients from the disordered range of health to somewhere within the adequate range of functioning, at which point therapy is assumed to have been successful. However, from the Biopsychosocial Therapy perspective, such a goal for change is limiting, especially for individuals living with chronic illness. Instead, the goal of Biopsychosocial Therapy is to achieve integration of the chronic condition as part of a healthy sense of self. Such an integration represents achieving the highest level of wellness possible while living

with a progressively degenerative or life-threatening illness. Fostering such personal integration and wellness is the primary outcome goal of Biopsychosocial Therapy.

3. *Constructivist perspective.* This perspective emphasizes the subjective manner in which individuals create or construct their perception of reality. With regard to chronic illness, patients construct or represent their illness in a unique manner, which may or may not be in accord with medical or psychological science. Nevertheless, this construction—referred to throughout the book as an *illness representation* or *explanatory model*—significantly influences their expectations for the process, goals, and outcomes of treatment and their adherence or compliance with a treatment protocol or regimen. Often this explanatory model—which can be thought of as the patient's case conceptualization—is at variance with the clinician's case conceptualization, and an important process goal of treatment is to negotiate and align these two conceptualizations or constructions.

4. *Comprehensive assessment.* Assessment that is informed by the biopsychosocial perspective is more detailed and comprehensive than traditional medical or psychological assessment. Using Biopsychosocial Therapy with individuals with chronic illness requires the elicitation and analysis of several assessment factors to understand not only the patient's psychological dynamics but also factors such as attachment style, health status, phase of illness, explanatory model, and so on. The purpose of such assessment is to understand the patient's basic pattern, from which a biopsychosocial case conceptualization and treatment plan can be derived.

5. *The primacy of relationship.* Effective work with individual complex medical or psychological conditions requires the involvement of the patient in the treatment process. Accordingly, Biopsychosocial Therapy emphasizes the establishment of a therapeutic alliance characterized by a collaborative bond between patient and clinician and mutual agreement about the goals and tasks of therapy. It encourages clinicians to assume the role of teacher and fellow traveler on the journey of integration and wellness, rather than expert and outsider.

6. *Integrative and tailored treatment.* An integrative approach, Biopsychosocial Therapy fosters the integration of theory and tailored treatment modalities and interventions. *Tailored treatment* refers to specific ways of customizing treatment modalities and therapeutic approaches to "fit" the unique needs, cognitive styles, emotional styles, personality styles, and treatment

expectations of the patient (Sperry, 1995a; Sperry, Carlson, & Kjos, 2003).

AN OVERVIEW OF THE BIOPSYCHOSOCIAL THERAPY APPROACH

The treatment process evolves in phases: engagement, assessment, intervention, and maintenance and termination; tailoring is essential at each phase (Sperry, 1999a, 2001b). In the engagement phase, the therapist endeavors to establish a working therapeutic relationship and to maximize the patient's readiness and motivation to change and develop. In the assessment phase, an evaluation is made of the patient's symptomatic distress and impairment, as well as maladaptive patterns of affects, thoughts, and behaviors. In the intervention phase, effort is focused on modification of maladaptive patterns and achieving some integration of the chronic illness within the patient's expanded self-conception, such that the illness becomes a part of the self but does not fully define the self. In the maintenance or termination phase, the focus is on maintaining the change and, when appropriate, reducing the patient's reliance on the treatment relationship.

On the basis of a comprehensive biopsychosocial evaluation, treatment is planned and tailored to the patient's needs, personality style, and expectations. Various psychotherapeutic, psychosocial, and biological or somatic interventions and strategies are used to implement that plan. *Psychotherapeutic interventions* include interventions directed at fostering internal change. These include cognitive restructuring of dysfunctional beliefs and related strategies to modify maladaptive schemas. They also include psychodynamic interpretation, fostering a corrective emotional experience, and specific intersession assignments, that is, homework. *Psychosocial interventions* include interventions directed at fostering better social skill training, couple therapy, family counseling, chronic-illness support groups, case management, family trauma care, workplace interventions, and family education (Fennell, 2003). *Biological interventions* include medication or referral for medication evaluation or management, diet and nutritional supplementation or referral for a nutritional evaluation and prescription, exercise prescription or referral for such an evaluation and prescription, and other stress management strategies, as indicated. Biological interventions also include patient education and disease management protocols, as well as self-management programs and protocols for specific chronic conditions (Redman, 2004).

BIOPSYCHOSOCIAL THERAPY IN CLINICAL PRACTICE

Four treatment stages have been noted to optimize treatment response and outcome (Sperry, 1995b; Sperry, Brill, Howard, & Grissom, 1996). The four essential stages are as follows: (a) engage the patient (and other provider[s]) in a collaborative relationship; (b) perform a comprehensive assessment and pattern analysis; (c) decrease symptomatology and increase functioning; and (d) maintain treatment gains and prevent recurrence. These stages are not unlike the phases of treatment that Beitman (1987, 1993) found were common to most Eastern and Western therapy systems and approaches. Rather, these stages have been configured and fashioned to the particular needs of patients and couples presenting with a complex of symptoms, functional impairment, concurrent medical or psychiatric conditions (such as characterological features that undermine or complicate treatment), unresponsiveness to treatment, or the presence of additional clinicians involved with the case. Three treatment tactics that relate to the third stage are also highlighted: (a) combining treatment modalities, (b) enhancing treatment compliance, and (c) incorporating psychoeducational interventions. Along with the four stages, these three tactics are discussed and illustrated in this chapter.

Phase 1: Engage the Patient in a Collaborative Relationship

Premature termination, treatment failure, and partial treatment success are often the result of inadequate engagement (Sperry, 1995a). Usually, this is due to the clinician's unwarranted assumption that the patient is ready and motivated to collaborate in the change process. Thus, rather than viewing engagement as the primary treatment strategy, the clinician proceeds with assessment and change intervention strategies and methods. Research suggests that when patients are not ready or willing to engage in a collaborative treatment process, noncompliance, partial response, and premature termination can be expected (Beitman, 1993).

Having two or more clinicians involved in the treatment process can further complicate the engagement and collaboration process. This occurs when one provides individual therapy and another provides another psychosocial modality—such as family or group therapy—or prescribes medication. This can occur because collaborating clinicians tend to have different treatment focuses and goals and relate to the patient differently in terms of duration and frequency of sessions. Whereas the prescribing clinician may be focused principally on managing relationships with the patient to maximize medication compliance and, with all hope, increase a positive placebo response, the nonmedical therapist is focused principally on enhancing the patient's self-management and interpersonal relationship functioning. Often, the two collaborating clinicians will differ in gender, age, interpersonal style, professional discipline, and attitudes toward somatic and psychosocial therapies. It is not surprising that the treatment process can be quite complicated, and interactional phenomena such as projective identification and splitting are commonplace.

Active and purposeful collaboration among the clinicians and the patient are essential not only to facilitate engagement but also for overall treatment efficacy. When the roles of both clinicians are clearly distinguished, frequent discussions about the patient and treatment goals can facilitate treatment outcomes (Woodward, Duckworth, & Gutheil, 1993). The quality of clinician–clinician collaboration is crucial to treatment, and mutual respect, trust, and openness are necessary in developing an effective collaboration. Collaborative communication is useful in sensitizing each other to their concerns. For instance, because the nonprescribing clinician sees the patient more frequently, he or she should be able to recognize early signs of hypomania in a patient who is taking an antimanic medication. Or the prescribing clinician, concerned that a patient's irritability might be a side effect of fluoxetine (Prozac), can learn from the other clinician that the patient is usually irritable.

Clinician's Role

What is the preferred role of the clinician in working with individuals who are chronically ill? Assuming the role of "expert," which tends to undermine the therapeutic alliance with the patient, is likely to reduce the patient's motivation for self-management and treatment compliance. Instead, Fennell (2003) proposed the role "fellow traveler." This role does not diminish clinicians' experience and technical experience, but rather it acknowledges that the patients have to undertake a long and arduous journey to integrate their chronic illness within their lives. It may be all but impossible to make this journey without the company and guidance of a clinician who may or may not be able to relate directly to the patient's personal experience of illness but who nevertheless is invested in the process. As Fennell (2003) discussed,

> The patient progresses, typically encountering cycles of adversity or suffering and then remission, and the clinician shares the experience. Instead of trying to dampen intrinsic and necessary countertransference reactions as undesirable responses, the clinician continually reacts and feels and pays attention to these responses. By using countertransference effectively, the clinician can actual enlarge and enhance the treatment process for everyone concerned. (p. 37)

Countertransference

Countertransference is a significant factor in psychotherapy (Gelso & Hayes, 2002), as well as in chronic illness. It is interesting to note that countertransference issues differ throughout the various phases of chronic illness. According to the four-phase model of illness (Fennell, 2003), clinician countertransferences are predictable over the course of the illness and its treatment. This section briefly sketches some of the common countertransferences that clinicians are likely to experience during these four phases.

Phase 1. Because crisis characterizes this phase, it is likely to stimulate feelings of revulsion, fear, and anger in clinicians. These feelings can arise in reaction to the patient's problem or concern, to the patient's efforts to deal with the problem, to what happened to the patient, or to what others have done to the patient. Other commonly experienced counteransferences are clinician's traumas, avoidance, overidentification, and failure to set boundaries. The patient's problem may trigger old traumas in the clinician's past. Countertranferential responses to patients at this phase may result in a clinician avoiding the patient by habitually rescheduling or missing appointments or unnecessarily referring the patient to another clinician. In addition, a clinician may overidentify with the patient and as a result become careless in setting appropriate limits and boundaries, both internal and external (Fennell, 2003).

Phase 2. Although some countertransferences characteristic of Phase 1 might be experienced in Phase 2, it is just as likely or more likely that conflict, normalization failure, and vicarious traumatization will be experienced. Either because the patient is slow to, or fails to, respond to the clinician's therapeutic efforts, conflict may ensue as the clinician becomes exasperated by the patient's failure to improve. Similarly, the clinician may experience conflict with the patient's family when it rewards the patient's nonhealthy actions or punishes the patient for healthy ones. In addition, clinicians may find themselves in conflict with treatment facilities or HMOs over various issues, such as failure to authorize continued care, and so on. Even though clinicians know better, they can experience a great deal of annoyance that their patients have not returned to normal. Finally, clinicians working with chronic patients can experience vicarious victimization at the hands of their professional peers who work primarily with nonchronic patients. Although these peers may find the clinician's work with chronic patients in Phase 1—who resemble acute patients—acceptable, they find the treatment of those in Phase 2 unacceptable and "sometimes regard clinicians working with these populations as choosing to work with undesirables" (Fennell, 2003, p. 241).

Phase 3. Generally speaking, the strongest and most upsetting countertransference feelings are experienced in this phase. This is because the work of Phase 3 magnifies distressing emotions that are experienced independently of particular patients. These countertransferences include the following: inadequacy, terror, depression, withdrawal, rejection, and resolution. Clinicians who are not fully convinced about the meaning and purpose of their own lives can feel inadequate in the task of helping patients explore their own life meaning and purpose issues. Facing such existential questions can arouse a sense of terror in clinicians. Or they may feel depressed contemplating the extent of suffering in the world. As clinicians grapple with feelings of inadequacy, terror, and depression in themselves, they may question what, if anything, they can possibly offer their patients. One way of "resolving" these existential considerations is to withdraw from their patients. Although some clinicians may refer their patients to a chaplain or spiritual guide, others reject the patient or the search for meaning, or both. Another way clinicians deal with these issues is to resolve their countertransference and find new meaning and purpose in their own lives, as they journey with their patients: "When clinicians openly acknowledge having questions and doubts of their own, they actually give significant aid and comfort to their struggling Phase 3 patients" (Fennell, 2003, p. 300).

Phase 4. The countertransference feelings and issues in this phase emanate from the success of the patient–clinician relationship. They are similar to those stimulated in the termination phase of formal psychotherapy. These include attachment, grief, loss, and pride. Frequently, clinicians experience a strong bond with patients with whom they have developed a productive collaborative relationship, and they thoroughly enjoy their company:

> Naturally, clinicians feel grief that this intensive collaboration is coming to a conclusion. They can suffer a sense of loss as their patients embark on independent lives. But clinicians also feel great pride. They have been witnesses to so much that their patients have endured. In the darkest times, their patients have courageously continued. They have believed in the clinician's faith that the process would work for them, even though they had little personal faith that it would. (Fennell, 2003, p. 337)

Phase 2: Perform a Comprehensive Assessment and Develop a Pattern Analysis

Functional assessment should include two patient characteristics that are predictive of treatment responsiveness and, hence, positive treatment outcomes: treatment readiness and explanatory model (Beitman, 1993). *Treatment readiness* refers to the patient's motivation and capacity to cooperate with treatment. Assessment of treatment readiness, and prompting and facilitating the highest level of readiness that the patient is capable of, is particularly important when psychotropic agents are the principal treatment modality. *Explanatory model* (and illness representation, both of which are discussed in greater detail in chap. 6) is the patient's personal interpretation or explanation of his or her disease and symptoms. This model can be fraught with misinformation or misattribution. Such "explanations" become the basis for patient education and negotiation. For instance, patients who experience bipolar disorder and believe that their illness was caused by insomnia and can be cured by a good night's sleep need to have their explanation corrected. Similarly, the patient who explains the experience of generalized anxiety in terms of a single early life trauma should hear the provider describe a more complete model of the illness, which also allows for these particular concerns about the early trauma. Specific irrational beliefs about illness or treatment must also be elicited and addressed. The delusional belief that the medication to be prescribed is poisonous is one obvious example. A less obvious irrational belief involves patients with low self-esteem. They may ascribe negative meaning to medication, viewing it as representative of their personal deficiency or worthlessness. This projected badness can then be externalized and dismissed by refusing to accept the medication and thus protecting themselves from further loss of self-esteem. Helping patients understand their illness is best done in a biopsychosocial context, particularly for those patients seeking the "magic" pill. Negotiated explanations that are tailored to the patient's experience are particularly valuable. Such explanations should be simple, integrate biological and psychosocial mechanisms, and incorporate some elements of the patient's explanation. For example, a man with schizophrenia may accept the fact that he has a biochemical imbalance that leaves him overly reactive to his environment and other people—the perceptual filter model of psychosis—resulting in social withdrawal and simple phobia. Or the patient insisting that hypoglycemia is the basis for his major depressive episode might be offered a treatment plan in which blood glucose would be checked immediately and reevaluated if a 4-week trial of medication is not successful. Finally, medication can be perceived as both a vehicle and an agent of control. It may be viewed as a chemical means by which the clinician exerts control over the patient's thought or action, and thereby, the patient's noncompliance is a means of controlling and defeating the clinician. Similarly, noncompliance may function as a projective identification, as when the patient's feelings of helplessness are projected on and induced in the clinician.

Although the current diagnostic system (i.e., the *Diagnostic and Statistical Manual of Mental Disorders*, 4th ed., [DSM–IV]; American Psychiatric Association, 1994) may have research and administrative value in specifying diagnoses across a range of patients, it is not clinically useful in evaluating patients for treatment planning purposes. In addition to the obvious problem of depending on somewhat arbitrary diagnostic categories and criteria, these criteria do not currently distinguish between symptomatic distress and functional capacity, nor do they address the matter of readiness for change. Clinically speaking, these factors are critical in planning treatment and predicting outcome. An evaluation model that specifies five dimensions is recommended: presentation, pattern, predisposition, perpetuants, and readiness for treatment (Sperry, 1995b; Sperry, Blackwell, Gudeman, & Faulkner, 1992).

Presentation refers to a description of the nature and severity of the individual's psychiatric presentation. It can include the type and kind of symptoms (i.e., acute, warning, or persistent), level of life functioning (i.e., self-management, family, intimacy, work, social, and health), past history, and course of the illness.

Pattern refers to the predictable and consistent style or manner in which a person thinks, feels, acts, copes, and defends the self both in stressful and nonstressful circumstances. It reflects the individual's baseline functioning. Pattern has physical, psychological, and social features, such as a sedentary and coronary-prone lifestyle, dependent personality style or disorder, or collusion in a relative's marital problems. Pattern also includes the individual's functional strengths, which counterbalance dysfunction. One way of specifying pattern is with *DSM–IV* Axis II personality traits or disorder terms.

Predisposition refers to all factors that render an individual vulnerable to a disorder. Predisposing factors usually involve physical, psychological, and social factors. Physical or biological factors include genetic, familial, temperament, or medical patterns, such as family history of a major psychiatric disorder, organ inferiority, family history of substance abuse, a difficult or slow-to-warm-up child temperament, or cardiac disease or hypertension. Psychological factors might include dysfunctional beliefs or convictions involving inadequacy, perfectionism, or overdependence, which might further predispose the individual to a medical disorder, such as coronary artery disease. They might also involve limited or exaggerated social skills, such as lack of friendship skills, unassertiveness, or overaggressiveness. Social factors could include early childhood losses, an inconsistent parenting style, an overly enmeshed or disengaged family of origin, or a family constellation characterized by dogged competitiveness or emotional surveillance. Subcultural, financial, and ethnic factors can be additional social predisposers.

Perpetuants refer to processes by which a patient's pattern is reinforced and confirmed by both the patient and the patient's environment. These processes may be physical, such as impaired immunity or habituation to an addictive substance; psychological, such as losing hope or fearing the consequences of getting well; or social, such as colluding family members or agencies that foster disordered behavior rather than recovery and growth.

Pattern Analysis and Case Conceptualization

Case conceptualization has become a core skill in cognitive therapy and in some psychoanalytic approaches (Eells & Lombart, 2003). Essentially, a case conceptualization consists of three components: a diagnostic formulation, a clinical formulation, and a treatment formulation (Sperry et al., 1992; Sperry, Lewis, Carlson, & Englar-Carlson, 2005).

A *diagnostic formulation* is a descriptive statement about the nature and severity of the individual's psychiatric presentation. Diagnostic formulations are descriptive, phenomenological, and cross sectional in nature. They answer the question "What happened?" For all practical purposes, the diagnostic formulation lends itself to being specified with *DSM–IV* criteria and nosology. A *clinical formulation*, however, is more explanatory and longitudinal in nature and attempts to offer a rationale for the development and maintenance of symptoms and dysfunctional life patterns. Clinical formulations answer the question "Why did it happen?" In short, the clinical formulation articulates and integrates the intrapsychic, interpersonal, and systemic dynamics to provide a clinically meaningful explanation of the patient's pattern, that is, the predictable style of thinking, feeling, acting, and coping in stressful circumstances—and it articulates a statement of the causality of his or her behavior. The clinical formulation is the key component in a case conceptualization and links the diagnostic and treatment formulations. A *treatment formulation* follows from a diagnostic and clinical formulation and is an explicit blueprint governing treatment interventions. Informed by both the answers to "What happened?" and "Why did it happen?" the answer to the question "What can be done about it, and how?" is the treatment formulation. A well-articulated treatment formulation provides treatment goals, a treatment plan, and treatment interventions, as well as predictions about the course of treatment and its outcomes.

Phase 3: Change Pattern and Achieve Treatment Outcomes

Decreasing symptomatology and increasing life functioning are the essential goals of all therapy systems and approaches. Individuals and couples who present for mental health treatment in symptomatic distress are seeking relief from symptoms they have not been able to reduce by their own efforts. Thus, symptom reduction or removal is one of the first goals of treatment. Usually, this goal is achieved with medication and behavioral interventions. According to phase theory, as symptoms increase, one or more areas of life functioning decrease; therapeutic efforts to increase functional capacity tend to be thwarted until symptomatology is decreased (Sperry et al., 1996). Six areas of life functioning that the Social Security Administration considers in making a determination of health or disability are self-management, health and grooming, social, intimacy, work, and family functioning. Along with levels of symptomatology, these areas of functioning are measured and monitored in current psychotherapy treatment outcome systems (Sperry et al., 1996). Most individuals who present for Biopsychosocial Therapy have problems with both symptomatic distress and functional impairment, and many have only partially responded to previous therapy, usually a single-mode, single-approach treatment. Thus, it is incumbent on the clinicians practicing Biopsychosocial Therapy to formulate a treatment plan comprehensively and integratively.

There are three treatment tactics related to this third stage that can ensure and optimize the likelihood of reducing symptoms and increasing functional capacity: (a) combining treatment modalities, (b) enhancing treatment compliance, and (c) incorporating psychoeducational interventions. Effective use of these tactics will increase the likelihood of positive treatment outcomes.

Combining treatments or *combined treatment* refers to adding modalities to the primary modality. When a patient begins a course of psychotherapy during which increasing symptoms preclude the patient from adequately functioning in relationships or on the job, medication may be combined with the primary modality. When medication is the primary modality, but medication compliance or the patient's safety becomes an issue, individual psychotherapy, group psychotherapy, couple therapy, or family therapy is typically added to the medication management treatment to increase treatment response and outcomes. It may simply be that group or family therapy is combined with individual therapy. Or, as in the first case example presented later in this volume, three modalities may be combined: individual therapy, family therapy, and medication.

Enhancing medication compliance is a major challenge facing both prescribing and nonprescribing clinicians. Key factors that are known to affect compliance include patient factors, provider–patient interaction, the treatment regimen itself, and family factors. The *placebo effect* refers to the belief and expectation that the patient will respond positively to treatment. It is operative anytime in any clinical situation, specifically when medication is involved. The placebo effect can be enhanced or triggered in several ways: by spending time with the patient, especially at the outset of treatment; by expressing interest and concern; and by demonstrating a confident, professional manner (Sperry, 1995b).

Incorporating psychoeducational interventions is a powerful optimizing tactic in psychopharmacotherapy. *Psychoeducation* refers to much more than merely explaining the medication, dosing schedule, and side-effect profile. Psychoeducation includes drug information sheets, patient education videos, medication groups, self-help organizations, support groups, social skills training, and more. Incorporating psychoeducational strategies and tactics in medication management is almost always essential to achieving symptom amelioration, particularly in the long term.

Phase 4: Maintain Treatment Gains and Plan Termination

Finally, maintaining treatment gains and preventing recurrence is the fourth strategy. Technically, *relapse* refers to a continuation of the "original" episode, and *recurrence* is the instigation of a "new" episode. For this discussion, both terms are used synonymously. To prevent relapse, the provider must assess the patient's risk factors and potential for relapse and incorporate relapse prevention strategies into the treatment process.

Therapists working in traditional psychotherapy with relatively high-functioning individuals with circumscribed therapeutic issues often find that such patients are able to achieve the treatment objective, maintain treatment gains, and successfully terminate therapy, cured of their condition. Clinicians working with individuals with chronic physical illness are less likely to experience such successes. In many regards, the situation is similar to clinicians and therapists who work therapeutically with lower functioning individuals with complex and severe conditions in which relapse is common, treatment is long term and open ended, and cure and termination are unlikely.

That is not to say that clinicians working therapeutically with patients with chronic physical illness never terminate treatment with successful cures. Cure and successful termination do happen occasionally, particularly when the chronic illness is relatively mild, when it is diagnosed early in its course, and when focused treatment and self-management efforts are optimal. Unfortunately, chronic disease tends to be less amenable to cure, and patients often do not achieve a return to normalcy. In such circumstances, both patient and clinicians can repeatedly experience powerful feelings of failure.

The reality is that chronic illness is usually experienced as a cyclic pattern of relapses and remissions, and often it is a downward cyclical pattern. Nevertheless, when others note improvement in a friend or family member who is chronically ill, they may conclude that such change is the start of a long, slow climb back to their prior health status:

> A single relapse may cause only disappointment or sorrow, but several relapses or even prolonged failure to return to normal can generate annoyance and anger in those who are not sick and varying degrees of self-loathing in those who are. (Fennell, 2003, p. 67)

CLINICAL INDICATIONS FOR BIOPSYCHOSOCIAL THERAPY

The clinical indications for the four Biopsychosocial Therapy strategies just described can be stated in both broad and narrow terms. In broad terms, all four strategies are indicated in instances when an adult patient or a couple (a) exhibits significant symptomatic distress or considerable functional impairment, particularly when biological factors are implicated—as in most severe Axis I disorders; (b) has a concurrent Axis I, II, or III condition that complicates treatment; (c) has not responded to a single-modality or single-approach treatment; or (d) is being provided treatment by more than one clinician. In narrow terms, each of the four strategies has more specific indications and contraindications—particularly the three tactics associated with the third strategy. Space precludes a detailing of them here.

PROCESS AND OUTCOME GOALS WITH CHRONIC ILLNESS PATIENTS

Planning and implementing treatment can be conceptualized in terms of process goals and outcome goals. As used here, *process goals* refers to specific procedural objectives and processes associated with each stage of the treatment process—that is, *engagement goals* of establishing and maintaining a therapeutic alliance—and *outcome goals* refers to treatment outcome targets for change that are specified for each phase of chronic illness—that is, to help the patient manage the crisis and trauma associated with Phase 1 of his or her chronic illness.

Process Goals in Chronic Illness

The Biopsychosocial Therapy approach specifies four treatment phases: engagement, pattern recognition and analysis, pattern change, and pattern maintenance and termination. Four sets of process goals are associated with these phases.

Phase 1: Engagement

Typically, four process goals related to this phase of treatment can be described. These are as follows: (a) establish a therapeutic alliance attending to tasks, goals, and bond; (b) maintain and bolster the therapeutic alliance; (c) repair ruptures to the alliance; and (d) recognize, use, and manage clinician countertransferences.

Phase 2: Pattern Recognition and Analysis

Generally speaking, there are four process goals related to this phase of treatment. These are as follows: (a) complete a comprehensive biopyschosocial assessment; (b) on the basis of the assessment, specify a diagnostic formulation; (c) create a clinical formulation, using the pattern analysis strategy; and (d) develop a treatment formulation with a plan for incorporating and sequencing the specified treatment interventions.

Phase 3: Pattern Change

Usually, three process goals related to this phase of treatment can be described. They are as follows: (a) implement the treatment formulation and intervention sequencing plan; (b) monitor outcome goals by phase of the illness, and revise the treatment formulation or plan accordingly; and (c) deal with countertransferences and other process factors as they arise.

Phase 4: Pattern Maintenance and Termination

Up to four process goals are associated with this phase of treatment. They are as follows: (a) with the patient, develop a relapse prevention plan; (b) process relapses as they occur; (c) monitor process goals, treatment outcome goals and objectives achieved, and other changes achieved; and (d) evaluate the need for a planned termination strategy, and implement it when appropriate.

Outcome Goals in Chronic Illness

In addition to these fours sets of process goals, four outcome goals and associated treatment issues encountered in the treatment of chronic illness have been noted. These are specified by phase of illness (Fennell, 2003).

Phase 1

The overall outcome goal is to help patients manage the crisis and trauma of being diagnosed with a chronic illness. At this point, patients believe that their illness originates entirely outside themselves. Significant treatment issues include dealing with their self-pathologizing and shame for bringing the disease condition on themselves, as well as their assumption that the treatment will be controlled entirely by others, making them feel even more helpless.

Phase 2

The overall outcome goal of this phase is to assist patients in stabilizing and initially restructuring their activities to match the limitations of their illness. Key treatment issues of this phase include helping patients develop self-observational, monitoring, and analytic skills relative to their symptoms and energy level and maintaining balance in four life spheres: personal maintenance, self-fulfillment, social and family relations, and work. Interventions to help the significant other and family members come to terms with new roles and expectations associated with the illness are required. Assuming that the patient is able to continue working, interventions involving the patient's supervisor and workplace accommodation usually are necessary.

Phase 3

The overall clinical goal is to assist patients in finding new purpose and meaning in life and constructing a new self. Significant treatment issues of this phase include facilitating their process of grief resulting from the loss of their precrisis self-conception and assisting them in finding spiritual or philosophical life meaning. Clinicians may also support the patient's self-management efforts and help the patient, significant other, and family to maintain their own case management. If needed, the clinician might support workplace accommodation or job separation efforts or might provide guidance about applying for disability benefits.

Phase 4

The overall clinical goal is to help integrate patients' suffering in their lives in a meaningful and sustaining manner. Key treatment issues of this phase include ensuring that desired elements of a patient's precrisis self are integrated into his or her newly constructed self. Other treatment issues include working with patients to develop a relapse prevention plan. This includes reviewing their skills in anticipating stressors and crises and monitoring their symptoms and health care needs, their self-management regimen, and how well their significant others and family members understand ways of ensuring their roles in the maintenance process. A final treatment issue involves the extension of life purpose and meaning. Whereas in Phase 3 this involved a "vertical' search for meaning, here the effort is more "horizontal," that is, extending meaning to everyday activities, challenges, and relationships.

CONCLUDING NOTE

This chapter has provided the reader with an overview of the Biopsychosocial Therapy approach—including its history, theoretical premises, and context—as it is applicable to working therapeutically with individuals experiencing chronic illness. An overview of the four phases of treatment of the Biopsychosocial Therapy approach was described and juxtaposed in a number of ways with the four phases of the patient's experience of chronic illness (Fennell, 2003). One of the basic premises of this approach is that a comprehensive, biopsychosocial assessment is essential to developing a biopsychosocial case conceptualization and plan for sequencing and implementing treatment interventions. The next chapter, chapter 6, details this assessment and case conceptualization process.

6

BIOPSYCHOSOCIAL THERAPY: ASSESSMENT AND CASE CONCEPTUALIZATION

A middle-aged female patient with a long history of diabetes is referred to a clinical psychologist by her primary care physician for smoking cessation. Because she had been unsuccessful in using a nicotine patch, her physicians had prescribed her a medication that can reduce nicotine craving but is also used as an antidepressant. The psychologist starts her on a 10-session behavioral smoking cessation treatment program. Unfortunately, she did not attend the second session and cannot be reached by phone. Two weeks later, he is contacted by the referring physician, who states that the patient is still smoking, has quit the smoking cessation program, and wants a prescription refill. The physician wonders why she wants the antidepressant if she is not involved in the behavioral treatment.

An adequate response to the physician's query would require a review of the initial assessment (Mamby, 2004). Did the psychologist assess the patient for the presence of early childhood abuse or neglect and for whether she was experiencing any symptoms related to trauma? Did he elicit her explanatory model about her diabetes and her smoking? Did he evaluate her level of readiness for treatment, her self-capacities, her level of family competence

115

and support, and the phase of her illness? The downside of not doing a comprehensive biopsychosocial assessment of a patient who is chronically ill is that it is difficult to predict and explain treatment noncompliance and disappointing clinical outcomes, as is manifest in this case example. Even though the referral was for direct treatment of the patient's diabetes, any treatment involving this patient—no matter how circumscribed, that is, smoking cessation—requires a complete, comprehensive assessment.

As noted in chapter 5, a comprehensive biopsychosocial assessment resulting in a biopsychosocial case conceptualization and treatment plan is essential in using Biopsychosocial Therapy in the treatment of chronic illness. That assessment process is highlighted in this chapter. At the heart of the assessment process is an extended consultation session, which consists of a semistructured assessment interview and some trial interventions. The purpose of the assessment interview is to elicit essential information about the patient's illness and its context, its perceived causes, and its progression and impact, as well as information about the patient's capacity and readiness for change. Then, on the basis of this comprehensive assessment, a biopsychosocial case conceptualization and treatment plan should emerge that not only specifies goals and interventions but sequences them to maximize the treatment outcomes achieved.

This chapter focuses on several key factors of the patient's experience of, and response to, his or her chronic illness. It details the key factors that are both useful predictors and markers of the patient's responsivity to treatment efforts. It also describes some commonly available self-report inventories that are useful adjuncts in the assessment process. Then it describes a method for developing a biopsychosocial case conceptualization and treatment plan. A case example illustrates this method.

THE ASSESSMENT PROCESS IN CHRONIC ILLNESS

Over the years, I have found that an assessment of chronic illness must be comprehensive, meaning that it must focus on biological, psychological, and sociocultural dynamics and determinants of the disease–illness process. Through trial and error, I have also found that it is best accomplished by means of semistructured interview, so that all pertinent dynamics and determinants are formally and adequate addressed. In addition, I have found that 13 or so key markers capture these illness dynamics and determinants. Exhibit 6.1 lists these 13 key assessment markers. This section describes each of these markers.

Disease Course and Progression and the Impact of the Illness on Functioning

The course or trajectory of a chronic disease can defy easy characterization. Nevertheless, it is useful to assess the course, progression, and impact of

EXHIBIT 6.1
Thirteen Key Markers in a Comprehensive Assessment

Disease progression and impact of illness on functioning.
Illness representation or explanatory model.
Adequacy of health behaviors and exposure history.
Early parental bond and adverse childhood experiences.
Personal schemas and family narratives.
Personality style or disorder.
Family competence level and style.
Religious and spiritual beliefs.
Patient resources and self-capacities.
Readiness for treatment and capacity for self-management.
Adequacy of treatment relationship with previous providers.
Alignment between clinician–patient explanatory models and treatment goals.
Phase of illness.

the disease. Some disease processes take a progressive debilitating course, whereas others follow a course that is mild and relatively stable with only occasional periods of exacerbation. Nevertheless, it is possible to consider the course of a disease state as mild and stable, moderate with a waxing and waning course, or progressively deteriorating and debilitating. Similarly, the progression of a disease state can also be described as early or advanced. Because illness is the subjective experience of a disease state, the impact of a progressively debilitating disease may be minimal for some individuals, whereas a mild and stable condition may significantly and negatively impact another individual. This variability of response means that clinicians need to accurately note the course, progression, and impact.

Illness Representation and Explanatory Model

Clinicians regularly observe that two patients with the same chronic disease and the same degree of severity will have markedly different psychological reactions to their illness and compliance with treatment. This variability of response has been studied by both medical anthropologists and social psychologists (Kleinman, Eisenberg, & Good, 1978; Leventhal, Diefenbach, & Levanthal, 1992). Whereas some medical anthropologists favor using the designation *explanatory model*, social psychologists and health psychologists favor *illness representations*. Illness representation evolved from early research on illness cognitions, that is, beliefs patients have about their illnesses, which influenced their compliance with medical treatment (Leventhal et al., 1992). Leventhal et al. (1992) contended that illnesses are represented by the following five characteristics: (a) their label or diagnosis and symptom manifestation; (b) their received biological or psychosocial causes; (c) their time line; (d) their consequences, that is, pain, disability, death, and so on; and (e) their management or curability, and by whom. Interpreting symptoms that are experienced is the first phase of developing an illness represen-tation. This involves both a cognitive component of the significance of the symptoms, that is, a threat appraisal, and an emotional component, that is, fear, anxiety, or alarm. Coping or illness regulation is the second phase, which requires processing information, forming expectations, making decisions, and regulating emotions aroused by the threat appraisal (Leventhal, Levanthal, & Cameron, 2000).

For all practical purposes, an explanatory model is quite similar to an illness representation. *Explanatory model* refers to an individual's personal interpretation or explanation of a disease process (Kleinman, 1988). This explanation injects personal meaning into the disease process, which pro-vides individuals with a means of understanding the causes, consequences, and prognosis of their illness experiences. Various questioning strategies for understanding a patient's explanatory model have been suggested (Kleinman et al., 1978). In my experience, the following questions have been quite use-ful in eliciting a patient's explanatory model:

1. What do you suppose is causing your illness?
2. Why do you think it began when it did?
3. What's your idea about how this illness works?
4. What effect does it have on to you?
5. How bad do you think it will get? How long will it last?
6. What kind of treatment do you think will make a difference?
7. What do you fear most about your illness?

Research on illness representations supports clinical observations that discrepancies between patients' and physicians' views can negatively impact treatment. One study found that when there were large discrepancies be-tween such views, the result was a worse health status for the patient and a subsequent increase in health care use (Heijmans et al., 2001). Illness repre-sentations can be assessed for both clinical and research purposes with in-struments such as the Illness Perception Questionnaire (IPQ; Weinman, Petrie, Moss-Morris, & Horne, 1996) and its revision, the IPQ–R (Moss-Morris et al., 2002). These instruments are based on Leventhal et al.'s (1992) self-regulatory model. A number of quantitative studies of the IPQ have been reported, including some that examined the consequences of these percep-tions and beliefs on moods. One such study of individuals with rheumatoid arthritis (RA) found that patients who saw themselves as responsible for their illness reported significant increases in depression over time compared with those who did not view themselves as responsible. Similarly, those who believed they would experience significant medical consequences of their illness reported that they became very depressed compared with those who believed there would be only minimal medical consequences from their RA (Schiaffino, Shawaryn, & Blum, 1998).

Adequacy of Health Behaviors and Exposure History

All individuals engage in health behaviors that reflect habitual daily activities that impact health, such as eating and diet, exercise patterns, handling stress, driving and seat belt use, and support systems. The adequacy of health behaviors is determined by need or prescription. For individuals who are chronically ill with diabetes, prescribed activities may include following a specific diet, monitoring blood sugar levels, and so on.

Research has increasingly acknowledged the causal connection and moderating effect of environmental pollution and toxin and chemical exposures on various chronic diseases. For instance, researchers from the Columbia University School of Public health reported that 95% of cancer is caused by diet and environmental exposure (Perera, 1997). Accordingly, an exposure history should be noted in the assessment. A dose–response effect may be operative. That is, an individual with a chronic respiratory condition may be relatively stable when exposed to low levels of a toxin; however, exposure to increased levels—that is, a greater dose—of the toxin may significantly exacerbate his or her illness or response.

Early Parental Bond and Adverse Childhood Experiences

Attachment refers to the emotional bond that develops between child and parent or caregiver, which subsequently influences the child's capacity to form mature, intimate relationships in adulthood. The impact of the early relational bond with parents cannot be underestimated, because this patterning and organization of attachment relationships is intimately linked to affect regulation, social relatedness, access to autobiographical memory, and the development of self-reflection and narrative (Siegel, 1999). More recently, this bond has been linked to health and chronic illness (Schmidt, Wuetrich-Martone, & Nachtigall, 2002).

Positive perceptions of love and caring from parents, usually the most important source of social support for children, have been found to be predictive of chronic disease in midlife. In the early 1950s, inventory ratings of parental caring reflecting feelings of warmth and closeness with parents were obtained from a sample of healthy Harvard undergraduate men who participated in the Harvard Mastery of Stress Study. Thirty-five years later, detailed medical and psychological histories and medical records were obtained on 126 of these former students. Analyses indicated that 91% of participants who did not perceive themselves to have had a warm relationship with their mothers—assessed during college—had diagnosed chronic diseases in midlife, that is, coronary artery disease, hypertension, duodenal ulcer, and alcoholism, compared with 45% of participants who perceived themselves to have had a warm relationship with their mothers (Russek & Schwartz, 1997a). A similar association between perceived warmth and closeness and future illness was noted for fathers (Russek & Schwartz, 1997b). This effect was independent of the participant's age, family history of illness, smoking behavior, and marital history, and the death or divorce of the participant's parents. Furthermore, 95% of participants who used few positive words and also rated their parents low in parental caring had diseases diagnosed in midlife, whereas only 29% of participants who used many positive words and also rated their parents high in parental caring had diseases diagnosed in midlife. Because parents are usually the most meaningful source of love and caring for much of early life, the perception of parental love and caring can play a special role in promoting long-term health. The findings are consistent with the hypothesis that love and caring play an important role in healing (Russek & Schwartz, 1996).

The prevalence of child sexual abuse ranges from 15% to 28% in female participants and 5% to 15% in male participants (Finkelhor, 1994). Estimates of physical abuse are reported by about 25% of adults (McMillan et al., 1997). In addition, over 20% of adults report growing up in a household with at least one alcoholic parent (Felitti et al., 1998). Furthermore, it has been noted that many individuals have experienced multiple types of trauma, that is, sexual, physical, and emotional abuse. Because trauma functions as a cumulative stressor, it should not be surprising that the victims of multiple types of trauma are likely to experience more chronic illnesses (Edwards, Anda, Felitti, & Dube, 2004; Edwards, Anda, Gu, & Felitti, 2000).

The range of chronic illnesses related to these adverse childhood experiences of trauma is vast. Diabetes and diabetic symptoms have been linked to abuse in childhood and adolescence (Kendall-Tackett & Marshall, 1999). Adverse childhood experience (ACE) is also linked to heart disease and cancer (Edwards et al., 2004). Researchers have noted the link between childhood abuse and arthritic breast cancer in women and thyroid disease in men (Stein & Barrett-Connor, 2000). Family violence has also been linked to chronic pain, cancer, stroke, emphysema, chronic bronchitis, and chronic hepatitis (Kendall-Tackett, 2003).

The implications of early trauma and abuse on compliance with treatment regimens and adherence to health education and self-management programs are dismaying. Research suggests that an early history of physical, sexual, or emotional trauma is linked to poor adherence to medical regimens (McCauley et al., 1997), as well as to reduced effectiveness of health education interventions (Edwards et al., 2004). Women who were sexually abused as children have a higher risk for HIV, presumably because of their impaired sense of self-efficacy about safe sex practices (Brown, Kessel, Lourie, Ford, & Lipsitt, 1997). Also, research indicates that individuals with childhood histories of trauma are more likely to continue smoking after receiving diagnoses of conditions contradicting smoking, such as lung or throat cancer (Edwards et al., 2000).

Fortunately, there are some promising nonmedication treatment options. One of these is called *disclosive writing*. On the basis of an expanding line of research on the positive effects of writing about stressful events, researchers have demonstrated that patients with asthma and rheumatoid arthritis who engaged in disclosive writing experienced long-lasting improvement in their chronic illness. Patients in the experimental group who wrote for 20 minutes without stopping on 3 consecutive days about the most stressful experience they had ever undergone showed a 47% clinically significant improvement, whereas only 27% of control patients evidenced such improvement (Smyth & Stone, 1999).

Personal Schemas and Family Narratives

Schemas are broad, pervasive themes reflecting an individual's view of self and of others that were developed during childhood and elaborated throughout life. They develop in childhood from an interplay between the child's innate temperament and the child's ongoing experiences—positive and negative—with parents, other adults, siblings, and peers. *Maladaptive schemas* are enduring and self-defeating patterns that typically begin early in life. Although they can also form in adulthood, maladaptive schemas cause negative or dysfunctional thoughts and feelings and can interfere with accomplishing goals and meetings one's needs. Adler (1956) first described schemas and referred to them as "lifestyle convictions." Cognitive therapy has elaborated a treatment approach called *schema therapy*, which focuses on modifying maladaptive schemas (Young, Klosko, & Weishaar, 2003). Young (1999) has identified 18 schemas. Because they begin early in life, schemas become familiar and thus comfortable. Maladaptive schemas may remain dormant until they are activated by situations relevant to them. Needless to say, the stresses of a chronic disease and the demands for involvement in and adherence to treatment activate such schemas. Accordingly, a patient's schemas should be routinely assessed. The clinician can use early recollections (Clark, 2002) or inventory or observational methods (Young et al., 2003) to assess schemas.

Family narratives reflect the systemic schemas of a family. It is the narrative (M. White & Epston, 1990) or story line that reflects the family's basic beliefs, customs, and values. For example, the family of a midlevel executive with severe cardiovascular heart disease and hypertension espoused a heroic family narrative. In this story line, family members are expected to be highly successful and show their caring for others by defending against forces that are perceived as threatening the "integrity," loyalty, and cohesion of the family. For this family, the struggle is ongoing and costly in terms of relationships. The overriding belief is that women are to champion standards for achievement and morality and that all others must respond by being highly successful, loyal, and obedient or risk harm and illness. Among those who must respond in this manner, for instance, are the husband who continually endeavors to succeed, but never to his wife's satisfaction, and the oldest son who has dropped out of college and failed in most business and relational endeavors. Family narratives are derived from the patient's schemas, as well as from observation and inquiry about family beliefs and values.

Psychopathology and Personality Style or Disorder

The presence of an Axis I or Axis II disorder typically complicates treatment. Even if the patient does not meet the criteria for a disorder as defined by the *Diagnostic and Statistical Manual of Mental Disorders* (4th ed.; *DSM–IV*; American Psychiatric Association, 1994), the patient's personality style can and does influence how he or she experiences an illness and responds to the treatment process (Sperry, 2003a). Accordingly, the clinician must carefully evaluate both the psychopathology and the personality of the patient.

Major depression is the most prevalent Axis I disorder comorbid with diabetes. Depression is associated with both poor glycemic control and increased rates of coronary heart disease in patients who are diabetic. Fortunately, therapeutic interventions such as cognitive–behavioral therapy (CBT) and antidepressant medication can ameliorate this medical condition (Lustman & Clouse, 2002).

Personality style can be defined as an individual's enduring pattern of thinking, feeling, behaving, and relating to the environment in a consistent manner and in various social contexts (Sperry, 2003a). A *personality disorder* is present when a personality style becomes sufficiently inflexible and maladaptive and causes significant impairment in occupational or social functioning or results in great subjective distress. A personality disorder indicates the existence of a long-standing maladaptive pattern of attitudes and behaviors in the way an individual relates to, perceives, and thinks about the environment and oneself, and that is of sufficient severity to cause either significant impairment in adaptive functioning or subjective distress. It is not surprising that patients with personality disorders and with chronic illness are a challenge to health care personnel with regard to keeping appointments, complying with treatment recommendations, and relating to health care personnel. Assessment of personality style or disorder provides the clinician with information about the health–personality dynamics of patients with chronic illness. Treatment implications of the six most common personality styles or disorders noted in patients with chronic illness are described in chapter 5.

Family Competence Level and Style

Family competence is the technical designation for the level of functioning of a given family. Highly competent—healthy and mature—families show warmth, respect, intimacy, and humor, along with the capacity to negotiate difficulties and maintain appropriate, clear boundaries. Families with low competence—less healthy and immature—have problematic boundaries, exhibit confused communication, and either are overcontrolling family members or provide no structure or consistency (Beavers & Hampson, 1990). *Family style* refers to the manner in which families relate to one another. For example, in the *enmeshed* or *overly engaged style*, families emphasize extreme dependency as well as closeness and sameness in how family members think, feel, and act. However, *disengaged-style* families emphasize extreme independence, which is reflected in relatively little cohesion and consistency in how family members relate to each other (Beavers & Hampson, 1990). Healthier families tend to have a high level of competence and a style that is interdependent, that is, blends both the engaged and disengaged styles. Because it is not unusual for patients with chronic illness to have come from problematic families, it is incumbent on the clinician to assess for such family dynamics. More impaired families have lower levels of competence—that is, a Global Assessment of Relationship Functioning (GARF; American Psychiatric Association, 2000) score of less than 40—and styles that are either overly enmeshed or chaotic. Finally, it should be noted that divorce is not uncommon when chronic illness has become debilitating. Often, partners of people who are chronically ill cannot adjust to these changing circumstances and divorce the ill partner (Joung, van de Mheen, Stronks, van Poppel, & Machenbach, 1998).

Religious and Spiritual Beliefs

Religious and spiritual beliefs can significantly influence a patient's perception of his or her chronic illness (Fennell, 2003). It is not surprising that these beliefs can also affect the patient's decisions about treatment and can affect compliance. Patients may refuse to take medication because of their beliefs about what their medication or their illness signifies. For example, patients may be reluctant to take medication because they believe that their illness is a punishment from God and that they do not deserve to be relieved of their suffering. Sometimes, older patients hold two disparate beliefs. The first is that life is meant to be a struggle and painful at times and that enduring such suffering is redemptive, that is, makes them worthy of a heavenly reward. The second belief is that authority figures like physicians should be honored and respected; that is, they should not question or dispute their physicians' judgments. The resolution of holding such discrepant beliefs is evident when they are given prescriptions by their physician: They will graciously accept the prescription but have no intention of filling it or taking the medicine.

Patient Resources and Self-Capacities

Patient resources refer to those resources—both inner and outer—that the patient brings to treatment and that positively impact the treatment process irrespective of the patient's actual involvement and adherence. *Inner resources* include the patient's readiness for change, coping and personal or social skills, motivation, ego strength, intelligence, achievements, psychological mindedness, courage, and past history of success in change efforts (Sperry, Carlson, & Kjos, 2003). A past history of success in change efforts, such as long-term smoking cessation or maintaining an exercise regimen for several months or years, is a significant marker in that it is a good predictor of the likelihood that a patient will engage in and maintain treatment adherence. *Outer resources* are specific environmental resources that impact the patient, such as the patient's social support system, financial resources, availability, access to expert treatment, and even fortuitous events.

Often, clinicians who elicit a history of early trauma in patients with chronic illness believe that this information has little clinical relevance because they are not being asked to provide intensive therapy to process the trauma. The clinical significance of eliciting a trauma is that the clinician can focus therapy on very specific targets. These targets involve *self-capacities*—inner abilities for regulating internal psychological processes and experiences (Pearlman, 1998). Examples of self-capacities include the ability to regulate affects, the ability to maintain a sense of positive self-worth, and the ability to maintain an inner sense of connection to healthy and benign others. These capacities begin to be developed in early relationships with key attachment figures, that is, mothers. When the attachment figure is not attuned to the infant or is emotionally distant or physically absent or abusive, the capacities remain undeveloped. Underdevelopment of self-capacities is characteristic of trauma. It appears that such underdeveloped self-capacities are operative in the affect dysregulation, relationship difficulties, and somatization of patients with histories of childhood trauma (Haven & Pearlman, 2004). Accordingly, individuals with chronic illnesses who exhibit these characteristics probably have undeveloped self-capacities that will inevitably complicate treatment.

Focusing treatment more specifically on minimizing affect dysregulation, relationship difficulties, or somatization can be a realistic treatment target. Among others, Linehan (1993) provided a protocol for increasing affect regulation. Johnson (2002) described a focused protocol for increasing relational bonding and harmony when relationship difficulties reflect an insecure attachment style. Kellner (1986) provided a protocol for addressing somatization in individual and group sessions when somatization reflects alexithymia, that is, the ability to identify and express feelings.

Readiness for Treatment and Capacity for Self-Management

Readiness for treatment refers to the patient's desire and capacity for making therapeutic changes. Readiness involves three components: treatment expectations, treatment willingness, and treatment capability (Sperry, 1995b). Though related, each of these three is a relatively independent marker of readiness. Patients can have high, low, or ambivalent expectations for change, and these expectations may be realistic or unrealistic. Generally speaking, patients with moderate to high realistic expectations of change do change more than patients with unrealistic or minimal expectations. Treatment willingness reflects the patient's potential or likelihood for change. Normative stages or levels of change have been noted in psychotherapy and pharmacotherapy (Beitman, 1993). The stages are as follows: *precontemplation*—denying the need for treatment; *contemplation*—accepting the need for treatment; *decision*—agreeing to take responsibility and collaborate with treatment efforts; *action*—taking responsibility and collaborating in efforts to change; and *maintenance*—continuing efforts and avoiding relapse (Prochaska, Norcross, & DiClemente, 1994). Knowledge of treatment willingness or stage of change is critical in predicting treatment outcomes because patients who have accepted the need for treatment, who have decided to cooperate with treatment, and who have made efforts to change and maintain change are more likely to have positive treatment outcomes than patients who have not. Treatment capability reflects the degree to which patients are capable of controlling or modulating their affects, cognitions, and impulses. As such, they are psychologically available to collaborate in treatment, in contrast to patients who are continually parasuicidal or who engage in treatment sabotage or escape behaviors (Sperry, 1995b).

Adequacy of Treatment Relationship With Previous Providers

Therapeutic relationship refers to the quality and strength of the collaborative relationship between patient and clinician. Because the therapeutic relationship accounts for as much or more treatment outcome as the specific treatment method used (Lambert & Ogles, 2003; Wampold, 2001), the adequacy of the relationship is an important assessment consideration. Establishing and maintaining a treatment relationship is a critical task of the engagement phase of treatment because, unless the patient is adequately engaged, treatment compliance and treatment effectiveness will be limited. Markers of the adequacy of the therapeutic relationship include consensus on goal alignment and collaboration, empathy, positive regard, feedback, and management of countertransference (Norcross, 2002). A good predictor of the adequacy of the therapeutic relationship is the patient's previous experience with other providers.

Alignment of Clinician's and Patient's Explanatory Models and Treatment Goals

A patient's explanatory model or illness representation can be thought of as his or her personal case conceptualization. Often, this explanation or conceptualization differs from the clinician's case conceptualization. To the extent to which clinicians recognize and acknowledge a patient's explanatory model, they are better able to anticipate issues in collaboration and compliance with treatment. Savvy clinicians are not content to elicit and acknowledge a patient's explanatory model; they engage the patient in a process of education and negotiation for the purpose of achieving a collaborative case conceptualization, which results in mutually agreed-on treatment goals. Presumably, because of this meeting of the minds, treatment compliance or adherence is optimized.

Phase of Illness

There are various phases of adaptation that occur in chronic illnesses. Fennell's (2003) four-phase model of illness describes the events of chronic illness and the responses to it that typically occur at each phase. This model was described in some detail in chapter 1 and is summarized here. Phase 1 involves *crisis*, and the basic task for patient and clinician is to deal with the immediate symptoms, pain, or traumas associated with this new experience of illness. Phase 2 is called *stabilization*, and the basic task is to stabilize and restructure life patterns and perceptions. Phase 3 is referred to as *resolution*. Its basic task is to develop a new self and to seek a personally meaningful philosophy of life and a concomitant spirituality. Phase 4 is called *integration* and involves the basic tasks of finding appropriate employment if one is able to work, reintegrating or forming supportive networks of friends and family, and integrating one's illness within a spiritual or philosophical framework. Fennell (2003) noted that "without sustained guidance from a clinician most patients find themselves either perpetually in crisis (Phase 1) or in an endless loop between the first two phases" (p. 8).

PATTERNS OF RESPONSIVENESS TO TREATMENT

After assessing a few dozen individuals with chronic illness, it becomes apparent that there is considerable variability among these individuals, variability that will influence the course and outcome of treatment. On the basis of an assessment of 13 key factors, it is possible to predict the degree of a patient's responsiveness to treatment. From my experience working with individuals with chronic illness, there seem to be three patterns of treatment responsiveness: minimal, moderate, and maximal. Table 6.1 summarizes these patterns, which I have initially observed in patients with chronic illness who present for evaluation and treatment. Identifying a patient's likely pattern of responsiveness during the initial evaluation is critically important because if change is to occur—for instance, symptom attenuation, improved compliance, increased integration, and so on—the clini-

TABLE 6.1

Patterns of Treatment Responsiveness Based on Key Assessment Factors

Assessment factor	Minimally responsive	Moderately responsive	Maximally responsive
Disease progression and illness impact	Moderate and disabling	Mild–moderate and moderate	Moderate and mild
Illness representation or explanatory model	External, negative	Negative–positive	Realistic
Adequacy of health behaviors and exposure Hx	Poor; high	Adequate; some exposure	Positive; low exposure
Early parental bond and ACE (abuse or neglect)	Insecure; severe	Insecure; some abuse	Healthy, secure bond
Personal schemas and family narratives	Disability prone	Limiting	None, health prone
Personality style or disorder	Disorder	Style or disorder	Style
Family competence and style	Severely dysfunctional	Partially dysfunctional	Highly functional
Religious and spiritual beliefs	Negative; complicating	Negative–positive	Integrated and positive
Patient resources, especially self-capacities	Limited, underdeveloped	Some; partially developed	Very adequate; developed
Readiness for treatment or capacity for self-mgmt	Precontemplative stage; low	Contemplative stage; some	Action stage; high
Adequacy of Tx relationship with other providers	Poor	Adequate	High
Alignment of explanatory model and treatment goals	Low	Adequate	High
Phase of illness	Phase 1 or looping from Phases 1 to 2	Phase 2	Phase 3 or 4

Note. Hx = history; ACE = adverse childhood experience; self-mgmt = self-management; Tx = treatment.

cian will, of necessity, engage in differential therapeutics, which means modifying treatment goals and focuses or tailoring treatment interventions accordingly. This would presumably reduce likely sources of resistance and increase responsivity.

Thus, from such a differential therapeutics perspective, clinicians trained and experienced in CBT would be likely to make headway in challenging negative automatic thoughts and restructuring the maladaptive beliefs of a patient with a pattern characterized by a moderate level of responsivity, while finding such a therapeutic strategy to have limited or no effect on patients with a pattern characterized by limited responsivity. Because such patients inevitably are constrained by early maladaptive schemas and abusive or ne-glectful family narratives, schema-focused therapy (Young et al., 2003) would be more likely to have the desired therapeutic effect.

Self-Report Inventories

There are several paper-and-pencil inventories available for assessing various psychological dimensions of chronic illness. I have found four inven-tories particularly useful in completing a comprehensive assessment of pa-tients presenting with chronic illness. Data from these instruments nicely complements the data collected in the interview assessment outlined in the sections that follow. Because a patient's explanatory model is a key factor in conceptualizing a case and formulating a treatment plan, data from the IPQ can be invaluable, usefully eliciting aspects of the patient's illness represen-tation. Having the patient complete this inventory prior to the consultation interview "primes" the patient for questions and inquiries about his or her explanatory model. The IPQ, Pictorial Representation of Illness and Self Measure (PRISM; Buchi et al., 2000), Millon Behavioral Medicine Diagnos-tic (MBMD; Millon, Antoni, Millon, Mengher, & Grossman, 2001), and Multidimensional Health Locus of Control Inventory (MHLC; Wallston, Wallston, & Devellis, 1978) add specific information that might not other-wise be elicited from a diagnostic interview.

Millon Behavioral Medicine Diagnostic

The MBMD is one of several instruments developed by Millon and his associates (Millon et al., 2001). The MBMD is a revision of the highly re-garded Millon Behavioral Health Inventory (Millon, Green, & Meagher, 1982). Both are designed for use with patients with medical problems and are particularly valuable for those with chronic illness. The MBMD is a self-administered instrument that yields scores on a number of variables associ-ated with health behaviors and outcomes. Eight scales identify coping styles, six measure the existence of psychosocial stressors associated with illness, and six assess emotional factors that might be associated with psychosomatic illnesses or complications. The scales were designed to assess the presence of factors that have been shown by research to relate to health outcomes, for instance, chronic tension, recent stress, pre-illness pessimism, and social alienation. Several scales were designed for use with patients diagnosed with allergy, gastrointestinal problems, or cardiovascular disease. These scales compare the patient's responses with those of patients whose illnesses have been complicated by psychosocial factors or whose course of treatment was unsatisfactory.[1]

Illness Perception Questionnaire

The IPQ and the IPQ–R are useful self-report inventories for assessing a patient's illness representation. As such, they are valuable in understanding a patient's explanatory model of his or her illness. The IPQ is based on and measures the five components of illness representations of Leventhal et al.'s (1992) self-regulatory model. Accordingly, the questionnaire consists of five scales to assess (a) *identity*—the symptoms the patients associate with the illness; (b) *cause*—the patient's own beliefs about the cause of the illness; (c) *time line*—the patient's perception of the duration of the illness; (d) *consequences*—the patient's expectations of the course and outcome of the treatment; and (e) *control*—the patient's beliefs about controlling or recovering from the illness. On a 5-point Likert scale ranging from 1 (*strongly agree*) to 5 (*strongly disagree*), the patient indicates the degree to which he or she agrees or disagrees with the items. Sample items include "My illness will last a long time"; "My symptoms are beyond my control"; and "Family problems or worries caused my illness." A particularly valuable feature of this inventory is that it can be easily tailored to particular chronic illnesses by simply replacing the word *illness* with the specific medical condition experienced. Thus, this inventory becomes a Cancer Perception Questionnaire or a Diabetes Perception Questionnaire, and so on. The IPQ–R is the same as the IPQ, with modification of two subscales and the inclusion of subscales that assess cyclical time-line perceptions, illness coherence, and emotional representations (Moss-Morris et al., 2002). A recent version of the IPQ inventory is available (C. A. White, 2001, Appendix 1).

Pictorial Representation of Illness and Self Measure

The PRISM is a visual measure for assessing the intrusiveness of illness into an individual's life, that is, the perception of suffering caused by the illness. Individuals are asked to look at a small metal board and imagine that it represents their life, with a yellow disk in the corner representing their concept of "self," and then to place a magnetized red disk, representing their illness, on the board in such a way as to represent its intrusiveness into their concept of self. The total time for the assessment is usually 30 seconds or less. The distance between the center of the yellow and red disks is measured by

---

[1]The MBMD is available from Pearson Assessments, formerly NCS Assessments (1-800-627-7271).

the clinician and reported as Self–Illness Separation (SIS). The greater the distance between the two centers, the less the individual's self is affected by the illness, whereas the closer the two, the more the illness is perceived as intrusive. The SIS correlates very highly with the SF 36 short-form questionnaire, which is validated for measuring quality of life in physical and mental domains (Buchi et al., 2000; Gardner-Nix, Dupak, & Lam-McCulloch, 2004). Recent studies reported on the use of this assessment device with various chronic illnesses (Vingerhoets, 2004a, 2004b). Before the PRISM took the form of a metal board, a sheet of 8.5 × 11-inch white paper in which a yellow disk was attached at one corner was used, and a red disk was placed on the paper. Presumably, a clinician could use this earlier format. In short, the PRISM offers a rapid method not only for assessing an important marker of an individual's experience of his or her chronic illness but also for monitoring or tracking the patient's progress from session to session.

Multidimensional Health Locus of Control Inventory

The MHLC is an 18-item scale developed by Wallston et al. (1978) that assesses the individual's attributions concerning health outcomes. Given the importance of the cognitive factor of control in individual health behaviors, this inventory can help the clinician anticipate problems in the patient's progress. There are three versions of the inventory. Forms A and B are general-health locus-of-control scales and consist of three time subscales: internality, powerful others externality, and chance externality. Form C is intended to be used for a specific chronic illness; that is, the clinician simply substitutes the word *condition* with the name of the illness experienced by the patient (Wallston, Stein, & Smith, 1994).[2]

CASE CONCEPTUALIZATIONS: ASSESSMENT AND PATTERN ANALYSIS

Case conceptualization has become a core skill in cognitive therapy and in some psychoanalytic approaches (Eells & Lombart, 2003). Essentially, a case conceptualization consists of three components: a diagnostic formulation, a clinical formulation, and a treatment formulation (Sperry, Blackwell, Gudeman, & Faulkner, 1992; Sperry, Lewis, Carlson, & Englar-Carlson, 2005).

A *diagnostic formulation* is a descriptive statement about the nature and severity of the individual's psychiatric presentation. Diagnostic formulations are descriptive, phenomenological, and cross sectional in nature. They answer the question "What happened?" For all practical purposes, the diagnos-

---

[2]Copies of all the MHLC scales, including Forms A, B, and C and a scoring key are available free from Dr. Wallston's Web site: www.vanderbilt.edu/nursing/kwallston/mhlcscales.htm.

tic formulation lends itself to being specified with *DSM–IV* criteria and nosology. A *clinical formulation*, however, is more explanatory and longitudinal
in nature and attempts to offer a rationale for the development and maintenance of symptoms and dysfunctional life patterns. Clinical formulations
answer the question "Why did it happen?" In short, the clinical formulation
articulates and integrates the intrapsychic, interpersonal, and systemic dynamics to provide a clinically meaningful explanation of the patient's pattern, that is, the predictable style of thinking, feeling, acting, and coping in
stressful circumstances—and it articulates a statement of the causality of his
or her behavior. The clinical formulation is the key component in a case
conceptualization and links the diagnostic and treatment formulations. A
treatment formulation follows from a diagnostic and clinical formulation and
is an explicit blueprint governing treatment interventions. Informed by both
the answers to "What happened?" and "Why did it happen?" the answer to
the question "What can be done about it, and how?" is the treatment formulation. A well-articulated treatment formulation provides treatment goals, a
treatment plan, and treatment interventions, as well as predictions about the
course of treatment and its outcomes.

Case Conceptualizations: Therapists Versus Patients

Effective therapists are skilled at developing, eliciting, and negotiating
case conceptualizations. What does "eliciting case conceptualizations" mean?
Therapists-in-training are surprised to learn that patients have developed
case conceptualizations of their own. Although patients may not consciously
be aware of their conceptualizations, these conceptualizations are nevertheless powerfully operative in the treatment process. Effective therapists not
only recognize the presence of such conceptualizations but also elicit them
and then negotiate a common conceptualization with their patients.

What are these patient conceptualizations like? They closely resemble
the structure of the three formulations I have been describing. First, patients'
or patient systems' description of their presenting problem or concern, including their symptomatic distress and their rating of their impairment in
the various areas of life functioning, is analogous to the therapist's diagnostic
formulation. Similarly, the patient's explanatory model of his or her condition or presenting problem is analogous to the therapist's clinical formulation. Finally, the patient's expectations for treatment are analogous to the
therapist's treatment formulation.

Where the patient and therapist case conceptualizations usually differ
is in their content. Whereas the therapist develops a case conceptualization
based on a critical understanding of the scientific basis—that is, the biological, psychological, and sociocultural basis—of human behavior, the patient's
explanation is more likely to be based on a highly personal, idiosyncratic,

and uncritical understanding or theory of human behavior. Social psychologists refer to this phenomenon as *naive personality theory*.

Why is it important to recognize the patient's own case conceptualization? Because the greater it differs from the therapist's conceptualization, the less likely treatment is to be effective and the more likely noncompliance or nonadherence will be present. This can show itself in many ways: Patients may come late or be "no-shows" for sessions; they may fail to do homework or take medication as prescribed; or they may prematurely terminate from therapy, that is, drop out. For example, imagine that the patient's nonelicited explanatory model for panic symptoms and difficulty doing grocery shopping and other outside household responsibilities is because of "a chemical imbalance in my brain." Imagine also that this patient's nonelicited treatment expectation is for Ativan, "because it really worked for a neighbor" but not for "talk therapy." Then, imagine that his or her therapist—who is considered a specialist in the behavioral therapy of anxiety disorders and is adamantly against the use of tranquilizers like Ativan—comes up with a diagnostic formulation of panic with agoraphobia, as well as a clinical formulation of symptoms being caused by avoidance behavior, and specifies a treatment formulation of exposure therapy; that is, the patient will be trained by gradual exposure to feared stimuli—large stores and other open spaces. What is likely to happen? Probably, the patient will directly or indirectly reject the plan for exposure therapy: either directly by refusing to adhere to the exposure protocol or by premature termination, or indirectly by halfheartedly being involved in the early exposure attempts. Now, if this therapist elicited the patient's case conceptualization, the therapist could then provide the patient with reasons why Ativan and other medications in that class are only a short-term treatment with high addictive potential and why exposure is preferable. It may be that, after further discussion, both agree that a safer and more effective medication, such as Prozac—which has FDA approval for use with panic and agoraphobia—will be used along with the behavioral approach.

The effective therapist's task, then, is to elicit the patient's or patient's system's case conceptualization. This means eliciting presenting problems, symptoms, areas of impaired functioning, treatment expectations, and, particularly, the explanatory model involved. An explanatory model is the patient's or patient's system's personal explanation or reason for his or her problems, symptoms, and impaired functioning. In other words, an explanatory model is akin to the therapist's professional and scientific explanation for the patient's or patient's system's problems, symptoms, and impaired functioning.

Effective therapists are able to reconcile differences between what are often two differing explanations or conceptualizations. Reconciliation involves negotiation. This negotiation process begins with the therapist acknowledging the patient's explanation and the similarities and differences from the therapist's conceptualization. The ensuing discussion allows the therapist to educate the patient about his or her illness and clarify misconceptions about it and the treatment process. Furthermore, discussion of the patient's or patient's system's expectations for the treatment process and outcomes facilitates negotiating a mutually agreeable direction for treatment and a therapeutic relationship based on cooperation. Then the specifics of treatment selection can be discussed.

Reconceptualizing a Patient's Explanatory Model

How might a clinician go about renegotiating and changing a patient's explanatory model or illness representation? Let's take chronic pain as an example. It is not uncommon for patients who experience chronic illness to espouse a limiting explanatory model that is essentially a biomedical explanation based on their experience of acute pain. The downside of the biomedical model of pain is that it does not consider how individuals' thoughts and feelings influence how they react to pain, nor does it reflect the biological, psychological, social, and cultural factors associated with chronic pain but not reflected in acute pain. However, the "gate control" theory of pain is a biopsychosocial model of pain that offers an explanation of how thoughts and feelings influence the experience of pain (Melzack, 1980; Wall & Melzack, 1989). In this theory, the experience of pain depends partly on whether the pain impulse passes a "neurological gate" in the spinal cord to the brain. The more the gate is opened, the more pain is experienced. Normally, the gate is closed by large sensory nerve fibers that respond to pressure or signals from the brain. Chronic pain is believed to occur when injury, disease, or infection damages fibers that ordinarily close the gate. According to the theory, patients can gain control over their pain by regulating their thoughts and feelings through strategies such as affect control, distraction, relaxation, and exercise. It is presumed that such strategies close the gate.

Reconceptualizing a patient's biomedical explanation of chronic pain to a more biopsychosocial explanation can be accomplished by suggesting that patients think about the gate control theory as a more helpful explanation of their pain experience. Such a reframing reduces their sense of hopelessness and helplessness while increasing their sense of self-efficacy. C. A. White (2001) suggested that engaging the patient in a discussion about pain and then explaining the gate control theory is a good place to begin the process of expanding and modifying the patient's explanatory model of chronic pain. First, the patient is encouraged to explore links between thoughts and feelings and his or her experience of pain. This can be done by discussing situations in which patients have similar pain experiences but different emotional reactions or by discussing the circumstances in which they responded differently because of the presence of others or demands on them. Such a discussion sets the stage for patients to move beyond their purely biomedical explanation of pain. Next, the gate control theory is explained in simple, straightforward terms:

There are sets of nerves that carry information to the spinal cord about sensations such as heat, vibration, or touch. So, if you touch the table then the sensation is carried along these sensory nerves to your spinal cord and onward to your brain. It can be helpful to think of these nerve signals as messages that have to pass through a gate before they get to the spinal cord or the brain. A message travels from our finger, along the spinal cord, through a gate and onward to your brain. Pain messages have to travel through a pain gate before they are experienced by you as painful. We know that feelings like tension or fear can make pains seem worse. We think that this is because they keep the "pain gate" open. We all know that things like relaxation, distraction and activities make pain easier to deal with. This is because they seem to close the gate to pain messages. You may have had the experience of people rubbing an area that is painful and then find the pain eases—this is because rubbing sends competing messages through the gate. (C. A. White, 2001, p. 140)

Then the patient is queried about how the gate theory explains his or her own specific pain experiences. Finally, the clinician might help patients contrast the differences between acute and chronic pain.

PATTERN ANALYSIS AS A FRAMEWORK FOR CASE CONCEPTUALIZATION

Pattern analysis, including its intervention planning and sequencing strategies, provides a critical "missing link" between theory and practice. As noted earlier, *pattern* is described as the predictable and consistent style or manner of thinking, feeling, acting, coping, and defending self in stressful and nonstressful circumstances (Sperry et al., 1992). Pattern analysis is the process of examining the interrelationship among four elements or factors: precipitating factors, predisposing factors, perpetuating factors, and presentation factors, including relational response factors. In other words, a patient's pattern or predicable style of behavior and functioning reflects and is reflected in all four factors: precipitant, presentation, perpetuations, and predisposition. Although it may appear that predisposing factors such as traumatic events, maladaptive beliefs or schemas, defenses, personality style, or systems factors primarily drive one's thoughts, feelings, and actions, the contention is that both individual and systemic dynamics are a function of all four factors and thus should be included in a pattern analysis. Because pattern analysis includes all these and associated individual and systemic dynamics, it provides a comprehensive basis for developing and articulating a clinically useful clinical formulation.

CASE CONCEPTUALIZATION OF CHRONIC ILLNESS

Individual or family counseling or therapy that involves health-related issues and concerns can be particularly challenging for counselors and therapists. Too often the health issue either is ignored as if it had no place in the context of counseling or is given precedence over other family interventions. Health issues must be processed as any other issues impacting the family, but the timing and sequencing of intervention's are critical. Typically, the therapist will begin treatment by immediately focusing on the health issue. It seems counterintuitive to offer health counseling interventions last rather than first, but as the following case demonstrates, it is only when the impact of individual and family dynamics bearing on the health concern are recognized and effectively and sufficiently processed that specific health recommendations or changes can be addressed.

Case Example: Diabetes as a Life- and Relationship-Threatening Chronic Illness

Miguel is a 47-year-old married White male manager who was referred for a clinical evaluation and treatment following his release from the hospital after treatment for a diabetic coma. Miguel, who is mildly obese, has been treated for diabetes Type 2 for 6 years. It was hoped that his adult-onset diabetes could be reasonably well controlled with diet and exercise, but daily insulin injections and blood sugar checks became necessary when weight management efforts failed and work-related stress increased during the first year. Aside from this chronic medical problem, his health status remains stable. He is the younger of two siblings, his sister being 6 years older. Miguel believes he was an unplanned pregnancy and that his mother was not as emotionally close to him as she was to his sister. His father, who is also overweight and has Type 2 diabetes, was a sales representative who seemed to be gone most of the time on business trips. Growing up, Miguel reports having had a few friends at his school who shared his fascination with collecting baseball cards. Miguel did reasonably well in school and graduated from college with a degree in accounting. He worked as an accountant for several years at a large utility company, a job he found reasonably well suited for him. Then he was promoted to a midlevel management position 8 years ago. Although he enjoyed the status and pay increase, he has found dealing with personnel issues to be very stressful. In fact, job and relationship stress are key themes in his explanatory model of his diabetes. He married Janine about 7 years ago. She is about 6 years younger than Miguel and worked as an administrative assistant in another unit of the utility company. It was the first marriage for both, and neither expressed interest in raising a family. As soon as they were married, Janine stopped working to "live the good life," as she enjoyed telling her friends. She seemed to live for the cruises and trips abroad they planned for their vacations. Miguel enjoyed these trips, too, but mostly for the companionship they provided. During their courtship and first years of marriage, Janine had come to be the center of his life. Afterwards—particularly after his diabetes was diagnosed—Miguel reports that their marriage was "less comforting." Like his mother, Miguel complained that Janine had become increasingly emotionally unavailable, particularly at those times when his diabetes seemed difficult to control and he needed someone to look after his special dietary needs and so on.

A week prior to the evaluation, Janine told Miguel she "needed more space" and wanted a separation from Miguel "at least for a while." This prospect was extremely distressing for Miguel. The next morning, Miguel stopped taking his insulin and went off his diet. Two days later, he was found unconscious in the men's room at his workplace. He was rushed to the hospital, where he was diagnosed with a diabetic coma secondary to diabetic ketoacidosis, a life-threatening condition. He was in intensive care for 3 days, with Janine at his side day and night. Janine cancelled her plans to move out, at least temporarily, and agreed to nurse Miguel back to health.

Case Conceptualization

Diagnostic Formulation

In terms of *Diagnostic and Statistical Manual of Mental Disorders* (text rev.; American Psychiatric Association, 2000), Miguel might meet the criteria for the diagnosis of an adjustment disorder and V-codes of relational problems NOS and occupational problems. Of more value from an assessment and formulation perspective is the pattern analysis summarized in Table 6.2.

Clinical Formulation

Pattern analysis suggests that when Janine voiced her intention to separate from Miguel, he responded by stopping his insulin injections and going off his diet. The result was a life-threatening condition, that is, a diabetic coma. An evaluation of individual dynamics reflected Miguel's self-view as being needy and physically defective. His worldview is that life is filled with dangers and the unexpected, and although others can be caring, they can also be inconsiderate and hurtful. His strategy is then to seek comfort and safety, using whatever means and at any cost to him. Stopping insulin and diet constituted self-harming behaviors that served to draw Janine back to him and provided some measure of security, connection, and caring. In terms of systemic dynamics, two dominant themes were highlighted in the couple's narrative: comfort seeking and self-reliance. This narrative "permitted" Janine to announce her plans for separation when it seemed like Miguel's diabetes was becoming a nuisance to her. The problem for Miguel was that the more self-reliant Janine became, the less caring and comforting she was toward him. As with other couples, their narrative takes on a corrective pattern during periods of conflict. In this instance, Janine's decision to remain in the relationship and nurse Miguel back to health was probably influenced by the recognition that if Miguel died or became permanently disabled, she would not likely have the financial resources to turn to for comfort seeking and self-reliance.

TABLE 6.2
Pattern Analysis: A Life- and Relationship-Threatening Disease Complication

Pattern factor	Formulation/treatment target	Intervention/sequence
Precipitating factor	Janine's talk of separation	1. Partner coaching
Predisposing factor	Miguel's defectiveness and rejection schemas; family's comfort-seeking and self-reliance narrative	3. Schema work (Miguel) 3. Re-storying (couple)
Presentation response	(a) Miguel's diabetic ketoacidosis	4. Health counseling strategy
	(b) Janine's efforts to support	2. Partner coaching
Perpetuant	Miguel's schema; family narrative	3. Schema work (Miguel) 3. Re-storying (couple)

Treatment Formulation

On the basis of this clinical formulation, the following short-term and longer term treatment goals can be specified. Table 6.2 summarizes these interventions and their potential sequencing. Note that the numbering represents the order in which interventions are sequenced, that is, parental coaching is first and third, whereas schema work and re-storying are second, and so on.

Given that Miguel's health behavior, that is, blood sugar drops and diabetic ketoacidosis and coma, is relationally specific, that is, to Janine's talk of separation, and not generalized, a conservative treatment strategy would be to focus on the short-term goal of reducing or modifying this trigger. This could involve a session or two with Janine in which the therapist coached her to find ways to meet her needs in ways that reduce "triggering" future health crises [Intervention/Sequence 1].

Next, treatment would include individual sessions with Miguel, with a focus on his defectiveness and rejection schemas and some conjoint sessions with Janine in which the couple's narrative of comfort seeking and self-reliance would be addressed. Coming from the narrative therapy tradition, re-storying involves focusing on previously unexamined or unemphasized aspects of those experiences (M. White & Epston, 1990). The resulting story includes pieces of meaning and understanding that are new or different and that allow for a positive shift in the original family narrative. In this case, re-storying involved less emphasis on self-reliance and more on caring and connectedness with one another [Intervention/Sequence 2].

In addition, Janine could be coached about the value of showing caring and concern in Miguel's recovery without feeling that he would become a burden on her. For instance, a private-duty nurse might be engaged, which would allow Janine to spend some quality time with Miguel and leave some time for her to engage in other activities and get together with her friends. This effectively would replace her "either–or" with a "both–and" stance toward Miguel. Such a stance would further reduce triggering a health crisis [Intervention/Sequence 3]. Janine's receptivity to the both–and stance might fail if this intervention preceded work on the couple narrative.

Finally, health-focused counseling (Sperry et al., 2005) is directed at maintaining stable blood sugar levels and adherence to diet and insulin regimen. Attempts to provide this kind of counseling prior to partner coaching and focus Miguel's schemas would most likely have been futile [Intervention/Sequence 4].

Case Commentary

In this clinical situation, the case conceptualization did guide treatment planning and implementation. Janine was quite responsive to partner coaching sessions and work on the couple narrative, as was Miguel. The result was that Miguel's health stabilized and has remained stable for the past 3 years. Janine feels more content with her life and Miguel, and separation has not been a consideration. It is noteworthy that the pattern analysis provided a framework not only for planning interventions based on the clinical formulation, but just as important, it offered a strategy and rationale for sequencing the interventions. As was previously noted, many health care professions would find it counterintuitive to sequence and offer the health counseling interventions last rather than first. Had health counseling been offered initially, it is quite unlikely that it would have had the desired outcome.

CONCLUDING NOTE

Of the four phases of the Biopsychosocial Therapy approach, Phase 2 is particularly important in that it identifies the patient's basic life pattern and the place of illness within it. Identification of that pattern by means of a comprehensive assessment leads to the development of biopsychosocial case conceptualization that provides an understanding of the patient and a tailored plan for modifying that pattern, which presumably will result in clinical outcomes ranging from cure to stabilization, plus a greater degree of integration and wellness. Central to such clinical outcomes is the comprehensive assessment. In working therapeutically with individuals who are chronically ill, it becomes clear that, like patients in conventional psychotherapy, they exhibit considerable patient variability, which is reflected in their responsiveness to treatment. A comprehensive biopsychosocial assessment aids in identifying patients in whom responsivity will likely be problematic. It also should assist the clinician in differential therapeutics—that is, tailoring treatment goals, focuses, and methods to reduce potential sources of resistance and increase responsivity. Finally, because of its importance to the therapy approach described in this book, completing a comprehensive assessment interview is highlighted and illustrated in subsequent chapters. Chapters 7 through 9 provide examples of completed cases with extensive transcriptions of the assessment interview process.

7
PSYCHOTHERAPEUTIC STRATEGIES
IN CHRONIC ILLNESS

This chapter highlights the use of psychotherapeutic strategies with patients experiencing chronic medical illnesses. Often, such patients are referred from primary care physicians, medical specialists, nurse practitioners, or health care educators who have had limited success in achieving compliance with a treatment regimen or self-management protocol or for whom issues of grief and depression interfered with treatment.

A useful practice protocol with such patients is to schedule an extended consultation session, usually of 90 minutes or more, to complete a comprehensive assessment that includes the 13 key assessment factors described in chapter 6. Both patient and referring source understand this to be a "consultation session" that will result in either additional sessions for health-focused psychotherapy if therapy is indicated or a written report of recommendation if therapy will not be offered. I have found that patients are much less apprehensive about having another consultation than about "seeing a shrink to get therapy."

A case demonstrating the proper and optimal use of various psychotherapeutic strategies, including a comprehensive assessment, is included in this chapter, with an individual referred with a diagnosis of systemic lupus erythematosis (SLE), which can be a serious life-threatening disease. SLE, usually referred to as *lupus*, is described in some detail in chapter 3. This chapter begins with some background information on the case, followed by a transcription of the initial sessions along with commentary, which is in turn followed by a case conceptualization and a suggested treatment focus and strategies.

BACKGROUND OF THE CASE

Jenna P. is a 37-year-old married Caucasian woman with SLE who was referred by her rheumatologist, who specializes in "stress management" for SLE. The referral report notes that the patient "seems to put herself in stressful situations that exacerbate her condition and result in significant pain and fatigue." Her diagnosis, which was made 7 years ago, shocked her into sobriety; she had a long history of alcohol dependence. The shock was because her older brother had been previously been diagnosed with a progressively degenerative form of lupus. What was originally thought to be a work-induced back injury in Jenna was eventually diagnosed as SLE. Jenna has a 12-year-old daughter with her husband, whom she was briefly divorced from around the time of her diagnosis. They have since remarried. Jenna made the appointment and appeared on time for the consultation.

SESSION TRANSCRIPTION

Following are segments of the transcription—along with commentary—of a 90-minute initial consultation session with Jenna. During the course of this consultation, I have two objectives: (a) to complete a relatively comprehensive biopsychosocial assessment of Jenna's experience of her chronic illness and life and, on the basis of this assessment, (b) to ascertain the extent to which she might be amenable to, and helped by, health counseling or psychotherapeutic strategies. After introductions, the session begins:

Therapist: Can you tell me about your health and medical condition?

Patient: I was diagnosed with lupus about 8 years ago. The diagnosis came when I was working for a utility company. At the time, I was doing a lot of heavy lifting and got really bad pain in the back, and they thought it was a back injury. The doctors did a lot of testing, like MRI and CAT scans, and couldn't find anything. But my brother had lupus, and I know about it, and it sounded a lot like what I was experiencing. I hadn't been tested for it or anything up to that point. So I said to the doctors that they needed to test for lupus, too. So they did, and taking the results together with my symptoms, they came up with the diagnosis of lupus. After that, I looked back and realized that my symptoms really started when I was 18 and had my first pleurisy attack. At the time, I didn't know what caused it, but now I assume that it was because of the lupus. When I first got the diagnosis, I was really scared because my brother has a worsening case, and I didn't know what to expect for me. But in the last 8 years, my symptoms really haven't gotten any worse. And I've learned from doctors and from what I read that if your symptoms don't change much, the condition probably won't get worse. But for my brother, it's a different story. His symptoms have continued to worsen as he has contracted other autoimmune diseases.

Therapist: So you have SLE, or systemic lupus erythematosus, is that right?

Patient: Yes, that's right.

Therapist: What's your understanding of your illness?

Patient: How I understand it is that my immune system is overactive. So it attacks itself and attacks good tissue. I know that if I overdo something, my immune system wants to fix it and then the muscle gets inflamed. I know that when I'm going to do something like cleaning house, I have to plan not to do anything later in the day because I'll be in too much pain and be too tired. So I've come to learn what my limits are.

Therapist: So there is a cause and effect. And your theory of your illness seems to be borne out by your experience: When you overtax your immune system, your illness is exacerbated and you feel the results of it.

Patient: That's right.

Therapist: Why do you suppose that you have lupus?

Patient: Probably a couple of reasons. I guess it runs in families. I already said my brother has it. For another reason it . . . I think I've damaged my immune system over the years, and according to what I read, that allowed the lupus to express itself.

Therapist: I think I understand that. . . . So what is it like to have this illness, and how do you feel about it?

Patient: I think I'm more aware of it now, particularly because of my symptoms. I know that stress plays a big part. Stress exacerbates my lupus quite a bit. And, usually when I'm stressed, I'm fine, but when it's over, then I'm in a lot of pain. And I've come to accept it, and I know now what I need to do. Usually, I have to take a break and stop for a while, but that's hard because I am a very busy person.

These initial therapist queries elicit the level of illness progression and impact, as well as the illness representation or explanatory model. Progression appears to be in the mild to moderate range, with its impact being relatively moderate. Her explanatory model is in line with the current medical view, and she recognizes what she needs to do to modulate or control symptoms, but she does not appear to fully accept this responsibility.

Therapist: Do you consider yourself a different person than you were 8 years ago?

Patient: Yes, I do, but there are other reasons for that. [*Nervous laugh*] The lupus is one reason; another is because I'm in recovery from a substance disorder, alcoholism. And that also has changed the way I live my life now.

Therapist: Could you say more about how your life has changed?

Patient: Drastically. I have been in recovery for some 8 years now. I was actively drinking when I was diagnosed with lupus. And I said to myself, "I'll never drink again as long as I don't get sick again." But when I found out it wasn't going to be so bad, I kept on drinking.

Therapist: What changed your thinking and your behavior?

Patient: Actually, my family did an intervention with me. At the time, I was divorced from my husband and living alone with my daughter. My family was concerned about me and my daughter and my drinking, and so they did an intervention. It was my brother and sister and my mother, but because my father was still an alcoholic, they didn't include him in the intervention. At that point, I was ready to change. I sort of knew that it was going to come, and when it came, I heard it. It definitely changed my life.

The disclosure about the impact of her diagnosis on her substance use, her self-promise about not drinking and the reversal of that promise, and her family's intervention are noted for now.

Therapist: In what ways did it tangibly change you?

Patient: My husband and I got divorced. And then we got remarried, and we've been together now for 4 years. My relationship with my daughter has been very good. She is back to trusting me again, in that when I say I'm going to do something, she knows I will do it. And in the past, where there were things that I said I would do, such as go back to school and have all these dreams, but I never followed through. I would just sit on a couch with my wine and cigarettes. But I was able to follow up on my dreams. I quit smoking a year after I quit drinking, and I decided I would go back to school and follow my dreams. I did, and I finished my bachelor's degree and have started in the master's program. I've accomplished my dreams, and my life has changed a lot.

Therapist: It sounds like a lot has happened and you've made some big changes in your life. How do you evaluate and feel about these changes?

Patient: I feel very positive about myself and the effect that my life has had on those around me. I go through guilt sometimes about the way I treated my daughter when I was living alone with her and drinking. She was only 5 when I got sober, and she is 12 now, and I know she doesn't remember everything, but I know it has affected her. For example, my friends graduating with me wanted me to go with them dancing after the graduation ceremony last January. When she heard this, she was beside herself and didn't want me to go, so I decided I wouldn't. She knows I wouldn't drink because it makes her uncomfortable anytime I'm around liquor. That makes me realize how much of an effect I have had on her.

Therapist: Does your daughter understand chronic lupus and your cycle of stress followed by pain, resulting in you being unavailable to others during those times?

Patient: I don't know if she understands the stress part of lupus. I know she knows that when I physically overexert myself, then I'll be slower. She knows that certain things give me an upset stomach. There are times when I have had to say, "I can't do that, I'm too tired or have an upset stomach." But I don't want her to be upset, I don't want her to feel guilty because I'm in pain or sick.

Therapist: Are her fears, such as you beginning to drink again, strong fears?

Patient: Oh, yes.

Therapist: For many, there is a one-to-one relationship between drinking and exacerbation of lupus symptoms. So in one way or another, your daughter is showing concern for you.

Patient: Yes, I see that. When I'm not feeling well, she'll give me backrubs when I am sore. She doesn't like it when I don't feel well. She is really worried and concerned about me. I don't want her to be too worried. She knows the lupus will not kill me but that it will always be affecting me. She knows about my brother, who has a more serious form of lupus, and has recently developed scleroderma and Raynaud's and other things, and she sees that he has it a lot worse than me. She knows he's living his life very fully, so she's not totally afraid of it. So she's aware of when the lupus is affecting me, and she'll back down from her demands that I do something for her.

Therapist: So you get enough experimenting and you know that it's real; there is a connection between stresses in your life and the exacerbation of your illness, and even the possible progression of it. It is generally recognized that ongoing chronic stress in individuals who initially had a relatively mild, nonprogressive chronic lupus can lead to a progressively degenerative form. What's it like to hear that you can influence the course of your illness, that you can control your illness, so to speak?

Patient: I know that, but sometimes I have a hard time doing what I need to do to control the lupus. I feel that there was so much I was not doing before in my life, and now I want to make up for it. Yet I know I need to slow down, but I don't want to. So intellectually I know, but emotionally I want to keep going. But I also know that the stress I have now is healthier than the stress I had when I was drinking, if that makes any sense, because I'm doing positive things now. So I do get overloaded, but it's not like the stress before, which was more guilt and things like that.

Therapist: At one time there was a distinction made between distress, and negative stress, and eustress, a more positive form of stress. Unfortunately, that distinction is not supported by research. In other words, the central nervous system and immune system doesn't make that distinction, and the net impact is damage to the body. Would this be a topic we could talk about for a little bit?

Patient: Yes, sure.

Therapist: Can you look at your symptom of pain and muscle stiffness and give me an indication of their severity now? You can do that on a 1 to 10 scale, where 10 is *very severe* and 1 is *very mild*.

Patient: On a daily basis, my symptoms would be around 3 or 4. I could feel minor aches and pains, but I'm very used to that, and it doesn't bother me. But by the end of the day, depending on if I've been on my feet all day, it could go up to an 8 or 9. There are times when my hips get really bad, and I have to lay down. If I have to go someplace where I have to stand and not sit down for a whole hour, then it gets really bad. And I think I know that it's going to happen, so I anticipate the pain. So if I plan to clean my house today, then I just know I'm going to be in pain. By the end of the day, I'll be in a lot of pain. The next morning, I wake up and am very stiff and achy, but after I take a shower I'm much better.

Therapist: Let's take a look at impairment now. That's the extent to which you can function in various areas of your life, such as work, social relations, and intimate relations, and so on. In terms of overall impairment now, how would you rate it on 1 to 10 scale, where 10 is *very low functioning* and 1 is *very high functioning*?

Patient: I would say a 4 or 5.

Therapist: How would you rate your functioning at work when you were to doing heavy lifting at your utility company job?

Patient: It was probably worse, but it's hard to say, because I was drinking then. So factoring that in, I would say it would be a 6 to 8. It got to be really bad, and after a while, I wasn't able to continue working. When I got home, I wouldn't be able to do much of anything other than maybe make dinner. But I really couldn't do anything with my daughter. I was too sore.

Therapist: Impairment and symptoms are two different factors; they don't necessarily go together. Which has more importance for you, the symptoms or the impairment?

Patient: It's impairment.

Therapist: From what you said earlier, it sounds like your job and career have been impacted. Is that accurate?

Patient: Well, yeah, because I'm changing careers and will no longer be doing heavy labor, but in moving into the counseling field, work impairment doesn't mean as much as it would have if I stayed in my previous job. I don't anticipate the lupus will cause a problem in my new career. So I think it would be more the symptoms, because they can be constantly present.

Therapist: It sounds like it is the symptoms. Now, in terms of your symptoms, you indicated earlier that you had come to anticipate them. And then they had the effect that you had anticipated. Has it ever been different? Were there any exceptions?

Patient: None that I can think of. Sometimes it was just the opposite. I wasn't anticipating it, and symptoms got really bad. So I'd be walking and my hip would go out, and I would know that it was time to sit down. So, as I anticipated it, it would happen.

Therapist: Then your anticipation was realistic?

Patient: Yes.

Therapist: So let's talk about the beginning of that sequence. You engaged in activities that you scheduled, which are pretty demanding on your body. But your head knows that this activity level is not good for your body. So what is the explanation? Why is it that you go ahead with those activities anyway?

Patient: It's probably because I've made a commitment to do something, such as at my daughter's school, where I should be involved. I'm really overcommitted there, and I can't say no. So I plan ahead and make sure I wear sensible shoes and try not to be on my feet too long, so it won't be too bad.

Asking about the sequence is part of the pattern-analysis process, particularly connecting precipitants with presentation and beginning to "test" some initial hypotheses about predisposition and perpetuants.

Therapist: There are many possible explanations for why you may be over-committed. Would you like to hear a few?

Patient: [*Nods affirmatively*]

Therapist: One might be that you are not really accepting your illness, and you act like you were prelupus. Thus, you act as if you can engage in extensive activity and you will not experience the consequences of that overactivity, which are pain and muscle aches. Another is that you may want others to recognize your good and even heroic efforts. Or it may be that you have very high expectations for yourself. I've heard you use the "should" word: "I should do this or do that."

Patient: [*Silent, but nods*]

She seems to balk at this interpretation, so I back off a bit.

Therapist: What do you suppose is behind your volunteering or overvolunteering, even when you have very little available energy?

Patient: I think it has a lot to do with the way things were before I stopped drinking. Before then, there were things I wanted to do but just didn't do. And now I'm trying to make up for that. I have to show that I'm this changed person and I can do all these things. I sometimes think I'm doing all these things for my daughter. I'm making up for the things that I didn't do before for her. She's even said, "Mommy you're doing too much, you can't say no." When I was on two committees at the same time, the demands were so great, she said that she couldn't wait till this is over, because she was getting too stressed just watching me.

Therapist: So maybe the explanation isn't fully that you're trying to please others or make up for the past, at least in the eyes of others. What other explanations might there be?

Patient: Umhmm. Maybe it's because when I see other moms doing all that stuff and being really good people, and I guess I want that perception of myself as being able to do all that, too.

Therapist: Now, do all these other moms that you're comparing yourself to have lupus?

Patient: [*Laughs*] No, and they don't volunteer like I do; they only do one thing at a time.

Therapist: So you're comparing yourself to others who don't have a chronic debilitating illness. Is that right? That's very interesting.

Patient: Yeah.

Therapist: Going back to the first hypothesis about denial of your illness, might it be more applicable than you first thought? Maybe there isn't full acceptance of your illness yet, added to the fact that you cannot be the person who you once were or would like to be?

Patient: [*Brief pause*] Yeah. You know, when you first said I had the thought that I only accept my illness when it benefits me. [*Nervous laughter*] That's to say that sometimes it was all right to have lupus, like when I had my last job, which I hated. So it was OK that I had lupus and had to leave my job.

Therapist: Because it gave you a legitimate excuse to leave your job.

Patient: Yeah. And it took away a lot of my stress to leave that job. But I don't want it to limit me from other things I wanted to do. Then, my lupus wasn't so bad. It'll be fine. I'll just have to watch it.

Therapist: Yes. [*Pause*] What your daughter said was very interesting, "Mommy you don't have to do all this, you can say no."

Patient: Uhmhum. You know, when I started being very active in her school, she was really quite excited about it. She liked me being the Lunch Mom and things like that. But, now that she's 12, she tells me, "Mom, you don't have to be here all the time." Instead of doing things to be with her, I get preoccupied with the activity and not really available to her. And she doesn't like that. She says, "You're not really doing this for me."

Therapist: Would this be another instance of you using your lupus for your own gain, such as you did when you left the heavy labor job and can no longer tolerate?

Patient: Do you mean as far as my daughter is concerned?

Therapist: I may be totally off base on this, and please correct me if I am, but one way of looking at this is that you may be using your lupus as a way of putting yourself in a situation that really stresses you but at the same time gives you the appearance of being an able-bodied mom who doesn't have a chronic debilitating illness. In a sense, it seems like you're using your illness against yourself.

Patient: It could be, but I'm not sure I see that.

Therapist: Let's look for some other explanations then. There is something that is operative here, and it is not just being the kind of mother your daughter wants, because she is already saying, "Look Mom, this is not good for you." And it's certainly not good for her. Yet, there's still this push for you to achieve, to achieve, to

	achieve past a point that is good for you. There is something going on that may be so useful to you right now that you don't even want to think about changing it.
Patient:	For instance, this afternoon I didn't have anything to do. I was all caught up with my course work, and my daughter didn't have homework or any obligations the afternoon or evening, and I felt uncomfortable. I didn't know what to do with myself. I used to just sit and watch TV all the time. And now I watch TV, but I have to be doing something at the same time. I can't just sit there and relax. I don't know why I have to feel busy all the time.
Therapist:	How were you before you stopped drinking?
Patient:	Then, I was just a procrastinator. I would just think about all the things I have to do, but I would never get up and do any of them.
Therapist:	What's your fantasy about what might happen if you just sat there, just laid back, didn't have the book, or didn't think about any of the things that you might need to do? So you would just be lying back relaxing and letting your immune system and your lupus go into a state of remission. Because they are not in a state of remission when your body and mind are stressed.
Patient:	[Nodding in agreement]
Therapist:	Being in a constant state of activity, even if it involves positive behaviors, will activate your immune system, which negatively impact your lupus and produces symptoms.
Patient:	My fear is that relaxing is being lazy.
Therapist:	What's the worst that could happen with being lazy?
Patient:	That it would be that way again. That's the way I was when I was drinking.
Therapist:	And if you are so lazy, like you were before, what would that mean?
Patient:	I would be afraid that it would take away all the things that I had accomplished.
Therapist:	And if it took away everything, absolutely everything, you had accomplished, where would that lead you?
Patient:	Back to being that drunk sitting on the couch.
Therapist:	And if it was even worse than that, where you'd be lying drunk in a gutter, what is the worst possible outcome that you can imagine?
Patient:	That I'd lose my family.

Therapist:	And if you lost your family?
Patient:	I wouldn't be anything.
Therapist:	You wouldn't be anything.
Patient:	No.
Therapist:	And if you weren't anything, lying in that gutter without a family?
Patient:	[*Long pause*] Then I wouldn't be here.
Therapist:	You'd take your life?
Patient:	I don't think that it would get to the point of taking my life, but drinking to the extent that I did is suicide. My dad died of drinking. He definitely drank himself to death. So if I ever went back to drinking, that's what it would mean. Because if I would pick up a drink again, it would mean I would have no hope.
Therapist:	How likely is that to happen? On a 0-to-100 scale, how likely is that possibility? And how likely would it be that if you relax on a couch and allowed your immune system to go to a very calm state, how likely is it that you would lose your family and everything that is important to you?
Patient:	No chance. [*Laughs*] No chance at all if I let my immune system get calmed. Realistically, that's not going to take anything away.
Therapist:	So you're sure it's a zero?
Patient:	Sure. But not if I did it all the time. But if I did periodically, and let myself relax, it would probably benefit my immune system and lupus.
Therapist:	What if you did it more than just occasionally?
Patient:	It would get better.
Therapist:	How likely? How high would you rate it?
Patient:	It would go up to 30% or 40%. I'm not sure what my family would feel, but personally it wouldn't feel good to me, and I would start feeling bad about myself.
Therapist:	How bad would you feel about yourself?
Patient:	I would start to feel like the person I was before. I just feel I need to achieve things to show myself that I not that person who didn't do anything. If I didn't do anything, I would be proving that I was that old person and that this new person is just fake.
Therapist:	It doesn't seem like you have too many options. You're either going to be a hardworking, driven person to prove that the

other person is basically worthless, or you'll be that worthless person.

Patient: Yes. Right now that's how my life seems. I would like to find a balance, definitely, because the lupus is telling me I can't live like that. So I do see it as God's little sign that you better find some way to balance this out. But, uhm, I know I need to do that.

Therapist: How will you know that it's safe to be a little bit more relaxed and taking better care of yourself? How will you know that you can be in a relaxed mode without being an awful person?

Patient: I think it will be when my physical symptoms are better. When I can do things and don't have the pain, then I'll know that I've been taking better care of myself. I know I need to come to that point. This summer, for instance, I don't have that much to do. I'm not on any committees, and I told my daughter we would have a relaxing summer. I'm actually anxious about it.

Therapist: You are going to be anxious about it if that fear is still about 30%. It will help if there are some safeguards in place, such as recognizing and accepting your symptoms. It's an important sign that most people like those without lupus don't have to alert them to take better care of themselves. That sign is a silver lining in the cloud of your chronic illness.

Patient: Uhmhum.

Therapist: If we can now shift a bit to your earlier life, can you say what it was like growing up in your family?

This led to an extended discussion about her bonding with her parents and queries about a history of possible abuse or neglect, as well as family values and dynamics and religious and spiritual beliefs. She reported being physically and emotionally abused by her father from age 5 onward, and once when he was in a drunken rage, he said they never wanted to have a girl—just another boy. Her mother did not intervene when Jenna's father would hit or scream at her for not being good enough or doing well enough in school. Consistent with her insecure attachment style were her personal schemas. Her self-view appears to be that of being flawed but somehow superior and tenacious, while her worldview is characterized by demandingness and unpredictability of life and other people. Her family-of-origins values seemed to emphasize a high expectation for achievement, obedience, and privacy, whereas the family narrative is that even though life is unfair and demanding, everyone has to succeed or at least appear to be successful no matter what the cost. Religious beliefs were consistent in her early family experience: She imaged God as critical and demanding and mentioned a common saying in the home, "God helps those who help themselves."

Therapist: A while ago you mentioned your daughter's recognition [of] and concern about your illness. Is there some way you could accept her concern at the same level of value and validity as your symptoms?

Patient: Yeah, I do. Because her speaking up recently has brought it to my attention that this is getting out of hand. I guess I want to be more relaxed. I think that she gets stressed watching me be stressed, and I really like her to be relaxed and happy, too. Because if she's relaxed, I'll be more relaxed.

Therapist: So you have two markers of health at this point, and there may be others also that can be useful. What will those two markers do to the probability, which is now at the 30% to 40% level?

Patient: That'd bring it down.

Therapist: What will it bring it down to?

Patient: Probably 10% or so. Because there's always going to be that level of concern.

Therapist: What will be the break-even point at which you'll tip one way or the other?

Patient: [*Frowns*]

Therapist: If it stayed at about 10%, would that allow enough margin of safety for you?

Patient: I could live with that.

Therapist: Our time is coming to a close, and maybe in the remaining minutes we might say a few things about your personality style. There is a theme of perfectionism that has emerged from our discussion. One of the things we can consider if we continue to work together is to explore the pattern of perfectionism and help you better understand your fear of going from one extreme to another. Anyway, it's a thought I had, which may or may not be on the mark.

Patient: No, it's pretty close. I've had people comment just this past year that I that just have to get things perfectly right. So, I think perfectionism is my pattern.

Therapist: Before we go on and discuss the next step, might you have a question or a comment?

Patient: A comment. The markers you mentioned about my symptoms and my daughter's reaction are things I never thought about before, as far as having something to mark my stress levels. I don't yet have anything to compare it to and to look for. I think I need to pursue these things. I know this appointment was set as a consultation meeting, but I'd like to continue meeting with you if that's possible.

Jenna evinces a moderate capacity for insight and can tolerate clinical interpretations, cognitive restructuring efforts, and interventive interview techniques, for instance, scaling questions, strategic questions, exception questions, outcome questions, and so on. She also appears to have a moderate level of readiness of change, that is, she is at the decision or planning stage. Important among her patient resources has been 7 years of abstinence, and she appears to have somewhat adequate self-capacities, including affect modulation and impulse control, but less development of others, such as self-soothing. The session concludes with Jenna and me discussing a plan of regular scheduled sessions and follow-up appointments.

REVIEW OF THE COMPREHENSIVE ASSESSMENT

Most of the comprehensive assessment was completed in this 90-minute face-to-face session, with the rest taking about 20 minutes to review the referral report and make brief phone contacts with both her primary care physician and her rheumatologist. Both report that she has been able to relate adequately to them and their staffs. It appears that the potential degree of alignment between my case conceptualization (described in the next section) and her explanatory model is adequate and that she is amenable to my efforts to educate her and negotiate a mutually agreeable case formulation. In my estimate, Jenna is between Phases 1 and 2 of her illness, in what is called *looping*, wherein the patient shifts back and forth between crisis and stabilization (Fennell, 2003). I am hopeful that focused psychotherapeutic strategies directed at her illness denial that feeds this looping and blocks her from moving to Phase 3 will be effective. On the basis of this comprehensive assessment, Jenna appears to have a reasonably good prognosis for health-focused psychotherapy. Table 7.1 summarizes the key factors of the assessment. A case conceptualization and suggested treatment focus follow.

CASE CONCEPTUALIZATION: PATTERN ANALYSIS

The basic presenting problem is Jenna's noncompliance with treatment recommendations to reduce stressors that diminish her immunity and subsequently lead to exacerbations of her SLE. Although her SLE has remained reasonably stable over the past 8 years, with relatively mild stress-related exacerbation and periods of remission, there is no guarantee that the disease process will continue to be stable and relatively mild. Although her brother's SLE follows a course of progressive deterioration, it is not uncommon for cases in which there has been relative stability for a matter of years to shift to

TABLE 7.1
Summary of Comprehensive Assessment for the Case of Jenna

Assessment factor	Partial responsiveness
Level of illness progression and impact	Mild–moderate and moderate
Illness representation or explanatory model	Medically accurate
Adequacy of health behaviors and exposure Hx	Adequate; moderate exposure
Early parental bond and ACE (abuse or neglect)	Insecure; some emotional and physical abuse
Personal schemas and family narratives	Overly demanding of success
Personality style or disorder	Mild disorder: perfectionism, need to please
Family competence and style	Midrange–borderline; mixed style
Religious and spiritual beliefs	Critical God; "God helps those who help . . ."
Patient resources, especially self-capacities	Partially developed and somewhat adequate
Readiness for treatment or capacity for self-mgmt	Contemplative–planning stage; inadequate
Adequacy of relating with other providers	Adequate
Alignment: Cl/Th explanatory model and Tx	Adequate
Phase of illness	Loops between Phases 1 and 2

Note. Hx = history; ACE = adverse childhood experience; Cl = Client; Th = Therapist; self-mgmt = self-management; Tx = treatment.

a deteriorating trajectory. Because the course of this disease is unpredictable and is sensitive to compromises of her immune system, and because of Jenna's denial of her illness and blatant disregard for medical recommendations—and her self-management program—to better manage physical and psychological stressors, her conditions can conceivably worsen. A comprehensive assessment based on the 13 key assessment factors resulted in the following pattern analysis.

Pattern

Jenna's basic pattern, which appears to be operative and consistent across various interpersonal contexts, is essentially one of striving to be perfect despite being chronically ill. This pattern requires her to overcommit herself while denying her illness. The pattern is enacted or operationalized in the manner discussed in the next several sections.

Precipitants

Various biological, psychological, and social precipitants tend to engage her pattern. First, she has to have sufficient energy and experience few or no pain or muscle aches (biological). A relational demand or opportunity arises in which she can excel and experience as compelling, for instance, a request to be involved on a parents' committee at her daughter's school (psychological). There are others, that is, parents and school administrators, who can observe and recognize her efforts (social).

Presentation

Jenna's response to a demand or an expectation is to attempt to excel, for which she experiences an exacerbation of her lupus and then symptoms, for instance, fatigue, pain, and other indicators of reduced immunity (biological). She receives recognition and the admiration of parents and administrators, who perceive her as a most committed and caring parent (social). She experiences a sense of satisfaction and superiority that she can accomplish as much or more than other parents who do not have a chronic illness, and certainly not a dreaded disease like SLE (psychological).

Predisposition

Jenna grew up in a household in which her father was regarded as successful by outsiders but as an abusive and uncontrolled alcoholic, who reportedly drank himself to death, by family members. She appears to be genetically loaded to alcohol abuse or dependence and for compulsivity and drivenness (biological). Her bonding with her parents was insecure and conditional, and she experienced physical and emotional abuse by her father and emotional neglect by her mother. Perfectionist striving became her leitmotif, with a self-view of being flawed, but somehow superior and heroic, and a worldview of the demandingness and unpredictability of life and other people (psychological). Family values included a high expectation of achievement, obedience, and privacy. The family narrative is that even though life is unfair and demanding, everyone has to succeed or at least appear to be successful, no matter what the cost (social).

Perpetuants

Experiencing pain and fatigue was a tangible indicator that Jenna was a committed individual and parent (biological). She experienced a sense of accomplishment and superiority over her illness and over others who don't have an illness (psychological). Receiving others' recognition reinforced her striving further (social). Her persona of healthiness continued to reinforce the denial of her illness. It is important to add that, in addition to her personality dynamics, that is, perfectionistic strivings, cultural dynamics seemed to be operative in fueling her illness denial: "The chronically ill are rewarded for unhealthy self-care, behaving as though they were feeling well" (Fennell, 2003, p. 68).

TREATMENT ISSUES

Treatment Outcome Goals

To guide treatment, many therapists reviewing this case might come up with a list of treatment outcome goals. These might include some or all of the following: process her denial of illness; examine and modify her schemas about perfectionism; process her compliance issue regarding stress–immunity–illness exacerbation; consider the advisability of, or possibly embark on, processing the relationship between her early childhood abuse and her father's and her substance use pattern; and process the automatic negative thoughts that emerged during the session (e.g., "It's important to be viewed as productive and successful by others, irrespective of the personal toll involved," "Lazy people are bad people," "Work- and family-related stress is healthier than the stress I had while I was drinking, because I'm doing positive things now," and "If I ever went back to drinking again, I'd drink myself to death like my father").

These goals are certainly reasonable. The question is, Why a particular goal, and in which order should it be pursued? In other words, Is there a preferred sequencing of interventions that both optimizes outcomes and the time—in terms of numbers of sessions—to achieve those goals while reducing or limiting resistance? Millon (1999) makes a convincing case that the sequencing and timing of interventions are essential. Accordingly, the pattern analysis strategy advocated here emphasizes the sequencing and timing of interventions.

Treatment Strategy

Based on the pattern analysis, a treatment focus is suggested. Table 7.2 summarizes the interventions involved and their potential sequencing. Note that the numbering represents the order in which interventions are sequenced; that is, coaching is first, schema work, cognitive–behavioral therapy, and re-storying are second, and health counseling is third.

Given that Jenna's attraction to certain stressors is situation specific—for instance, situations in which she can overachieve and act heroically in view of others who are able bodied—a conservative treatment strategy would be to focus on the short-term goal of reducing or modifying this trigger. This could involve a focused discussion in which the therapist coaches Jenna on ways to meet her psychological and social needs that are not so costly, that is, triggering an exacerbation of lupus. It would also include modifying some of her automatic negative thoughts, including "Lazy people are bad people," and so on [Intervention/Sequence 1]. Next, treatment would include individual sessions with Jenna, using psychotherapeutic strategies to clarify, confront, interpret, and restructure her perfectionism and heroic schemas.

TABLE 7.2

Pattern Analysis and Treatment Strategy for the Case of Jenna

Pattern factor	Formulation/treatment target	Intervention/sequence
Precipitating factor	(P) Opportunity to excel that is compelling; (B) Sufficient energy and not distressed or in pain; (S) Others who can observe and recognize her efforts	1. Coaching on trigger reduction and modifying specified automatic thoughts (Jenna)
Predisposing factor	(B) Genetically loaded for compulsivity and substance abuse; (P) Insecure attachment and early abuse; perfectionist striving; (S) Family values achievement as measure of worth; narrative: appearance of success despite the cost	2. Schema work (Jenna) 2. CBT/Rx for compulsivity (Jenna) 2. Re-storying (family)
Presentation response	(B) Excels exacerbation of Sx; (S) Receives others' recognition and admiration; (P) Sense of superiority for accomplishing more than able-bodied person	3. Health counseling (Jenna)
Perpetuant	(B/P/S) Experiencing pain and getting others' recognition proves she is successful	2. Schema work (Jenna) 2. Re-storying (family)

Note. Letters in parentheses represent biological (B), psychological (P), and sociological (S) factors. CBT = cognitive–behavioral therapy; Rx = treatment; Sx = symptoms.

It would also include other sessions—including her husband and possibly her daughter—which would focus on re-storying the family narrative to one that involved less emphasis on the appearance of success at all costs and more emphasis on success in relaxing and developing satisfying family relationships [Intervention/Sequence 2].

Finally, health-focused counseling strategies would be directed at managing stress and adherence to her self-management protocol, particularly increasing her immunocompetence. Attempts to provide this kind of counseling prior to modifying her automatic negative thoughts, schemas, and family narrative and reducing her compulsivity would most likely have been futile [Intervention/Sequence 3].

TREATMENT PROCESS AND OUTCOME OF THE CASE

A follow-up appointment was made, and Jenna began health-focused psychotherapy. The initial treatment contract involved eight sessions, six of which were scheduled weekly and the last two sessions scheduled biweekly. Much of the first session focused on intervention/sequencing 1, and Jenna was helped to find other ways she could meet her needs without triggering lupus symptoms. The first session also addressed the negative automatic thoughts noted in the comprehensive assessment. Sessions 2 through 5 focused on schema modification, whereas Session 6 was a conjoint session focused on re-storying the family narrative. During these sessions, as the theme of accepting her illness was processed, treatment indirectly emphasized the goals of Phase 3 of a chronic illness (resolution). During this time, Jenna became a regular participant in a lupus support group. Some years earlier, she had attended a meeting or two before dropping out. Now she was ready to receive the support of others for just being who she was. Session 7 focused on the health counseling goal, whereas Session 8 focused on evaluating progress and formalizing a relapse prevention plan. Jenna had been reading Fennell's (2001) *Chronic Illness Workbook* and recognized that integration (Phase 4) was where she needed to be. We mutually negotiated a contract for follow-up sessions every 10 to 12 weeks, or sooner if needed. Two years after completing our eighth session, I had met with Jenna a total of nine times. She had been quite effective in controlling stress triggers and had reached and remained in Phase 4 of her illness.

CONCLUDING NOTE

This case example illustrates a typical first encounter of the Biopsychosocial Therapy approach to working therapeutically with patients with chronic physical illness. In addition to undergoing a rather comprehensive assessment, the patient is evaluated for his or her capacity to engage in health-focused psychotherapy and the likely prognosis. The example also illustrates a complete case conceptualization and treatment plan and the sequencing of psychotherapeutic strategies and interventions. In this case, on the basis of the pattern analysis, I concluded that it was absolutely essential for the health-focused psychotherapeutic strategies to be used prior to introducing health-focused counseling strategies to achieve positive clinical outcomes. Finally, it was noted that the treatment focus involved the primary use of standard or less intensive psychotherapeutic strategies. By contrast, in the next chapter, a case is described that illustrates the primary use of more intensive psychotherapeutic strategies.

8

INTENSIVE PSYCHOTHERAPEUTIC STRATEGIES IN CHRONIC ILLNESS

This chapter highlights the use of intensive health-focused psychotherapy strategies with chronic physical illness. Intensive health-focused psychotherapeutic strategies can be particularly useful in circumstances in which patients have responded only partially, or not at all, to standard health-focused psychotherapeutic strategies. Standard health-focused psychotherapy (cf. chap. 7) often involves the use of cognitive–behavioral therapy strategies with patients with chronic illness. These strategies include behavioral treatment methods, situational and environmental methods, and, particularly, cognitive treatment methods. Typically, the cognitive methods used involve identifying and modifying automatic thoughts, maintaining attentional control, identifying thinking biases, modifying maladaptive beliefs, and sometimes modifying schemas (C. A. White, 2001). These strategies are effective for many—perhaps the majority of—patients in whom health-focused psychotherapy is indicated. However, patients who have not fared well in such treatment and whom present with a more complicated picture—often involving childhood abuse or neglect histories and personality disorders reflected in early maladaptive schemas—are more likely to respond to therapy that focuses intensively on modifying those maladaptive schemas and patterns (Young, Klosko, & Weishaar, 2003). Other intensive health-focused psychotherapeutic strategies include interpretation, internalization (Binder, 2004), life-style analysis (Adler, 1956), and hypnotherapy.

This chapter illustrates the use of intensive health-focused psychotherapy strategies with a patient with a long-standing diagnosis of epilepsy who has not responded to various medical and psychological treatments. The format for this case is an extended consultation session in which a comprehensive assessment of the patient's illness dynamics, followed by an evaluation of her capacity for intensive treatment, engages the patient in an intensive therapeutic process. Segments of the transcription of this extended consultation session are provided, along with case commentary. In addition, a review of the assessment findings, a brief case conceptualization, and treatment recommendations are included.

BACKGROUND OF THE CASE

Kathleen Z. is a 29-year-old married Caucasian woman with a history of epilepsy who was referred by her neurologist for an "evaluation and treatment of a complex symptom picture, which is a problem largely psychological in nature." The patient has been married for about 5 years and has no children, although the couple has recently been discussing the possibility of beginning a family. She was born in Ireland and moved to the United States with her parents at the age of 5. She was initially diagnosed with grand mal seizures by her family physician 15 years ago and treated with an antiepileptic medication for approximately 1 year. A subsequent "attack"—as Kathleen refers to them—was evaluated by an epilepsy specialist, who was not absolutely convinced of the previously given diagnosis. Nevertheless, he let it stand, although he stopped her medication and suggested she avoid stress. Approximately 2.5 years ago, she reported the reappearance of "really bad attacks, one right after the other." She was evaluated by the referring neurologist, who favored a diagnosis of psuedoseizures. As a result, he framed her attacks as atypical panic attacks and referred her to a psychiatrist for medication evaluation and management. After his evaluation, the psychiatrist was not convinced that she met the criteria for panic disorder without agoraphobia but did give her the presumptive diagnosis of panic disorder NOS. He also prescribed an anxiolytic medication and steered her to a therapist in his office for "anxiety- and stress-management" training. A review of the psychiatrist's clinical report on Kathleen indicated the presence of "borderline and histrionic personality traits that are likely to confound the treatment process." Because pseudoseizures can and do occur in individuals with diagnosed cases of epilepsy, none of the physicians who evaluated or treated Kathleen were willing to dissuade her from the conviction that she had "only" an anxiety disorder. An appointment was made for an extended consultation, with the understanding that the consultation would result in recommendations to her and her referring physician and that health-focused psychotherapy might or might not be a recommendation.

SESSION TRANSCRIPTION

After a brief introduction, the session begins:

Therapist: Your doctor's referral report says you've been having some difficult symptoms. Could you tell me about them?

Patient: Well, I've had epilepsy for about 15 years, and a few years ago started having what you might call panic attacks for about 2 years now. Right before I got married, I was having these attacks where it would start coming up my leg and going into my arm. I would get like really, really tight, and it would go over to my left arm and then go down my leg, and they never could understand what the problem was. I've gone to see doctors. I'm currently seeing a therapist and a psychiatrist, and the psychiatrist says that these are panic attacks. But the attacks I get don't occur with a panic attack. I pass out and might fall and hit my head or something like that, and then I will awake, and I won't know where I'm at, and they say that those attacks are not related to panic attacks. I think I do get panic attacks, too. But the doctors just cannot pinpoint what kind I do get.

Therapist: So you mentioned panic attacks and epilepsy.

Patient: Right.

Therapist: In your mind, do you have one or both?

Patient: Um, in one way I think I have both, and sometimes I think I just have panic. I really wish I could pinpoint down what I have.

Therapist: And if you could do that, how would your life be different?

Patient: Oh, it would be much better. I wouldn't have to worry about anything, or, I mean, I know people worry about things. But I would feel more at ease with life, um, with being married and everything. I have to think of really if we want to have children, my husband and I. I would have to get off medication first or see if I'm well enough to have children. So that kind of is not worrisome, but it's on my . . . it's on both of our minds.

Therapist: So, if you could get clarity, whether it's one or both, it would make all the difference in the world.

Patient: Oh, much. It would. Because I would be able to enjoy life and be happy. Because I just don't laugh. I just sit there, and I'm like a bum. My husband says, "Why don't you laugh?" I said, "I can't." But when I'm away from him, because I volunteer at a hospital in the gift shop, I'm fine. I'm happy. I'm content there. It's like every time that I go to start a job, that's when it happens. I get panicky.

Therapist: A job, meaning a paid position?

Patient: Yes, a job.

Therapist: Not a volunteer position?

Patient: No. When I go to start a job, I get all panicky and then I can't work. And then my husband gets all mad with me, saying, you know, he says, "Why can't you get and keep a job?" He doesn't get violently mad. He just gets upset, which I don't blame him. He was going to college at the time when I was having these attacks. He was about to graduate, and he asked me, please don't have any of your attacks while I'm trying to do my final exams. And what did I do? I had panic the whole week of his finals. Oh, was he mad. But at least he graduated.

Therapist: How did he manage to do that?

Patient: I don't know. He just did.

Therapist: So, somehow he was able to take his final exams, and your symptoms didn't seem to make all that much of a difference in his life.

Patient: No.

Therapist: What difference did those symptoms make in your life at that time?

Patient: Well, we were planning our wedding at the time, and we had to cut the guest list from 200 people down to only 40. That's including myself and my husband. We had to. We said, Why have a big wedding and risk that on the wedding day that I might be on the floor with an attack? We'd have to cancel out and lose all the money, but if we just had a small wedding with a restaurant reception with our families, and then later have a big party at the house like for all our friends and everything. . . . It worked out, and I was so much better.

Therapist: Is it possible you could have had an attack at your reception whether there were 200 or 40 people?

Patient: Right, but I was fine that day. I was fine.

Therapist: What do you think accounts for that?

Patient: I don't know. I really don't. I mean, I think I was . . . see, if I don't think about it, I don't get them. So I probably had a lot on my mind where I said okay, you know, they just didn't even appear that day. And then the day we had our outside party, nothing happened that day because I was too busy running around making sure everything was in its place and all, and I was fine.

Therapist: Was that some sort of a rule for you that you noticed then? If you are preoccupied, if you have things that need to get done, then it won't be a problem?

Patient: Right. If I'm preoccupied, if I'm sitting at home all the time and watching TV, or taking naps, or just doing nothing, the attacks can happen. But if I get out and volunteer or go shopping and not buy anything, then things are fine, and I don't have attacks.

Therapist: That sounds like an ironclad rule: Be preoccupied, and no attacks will happen. Has that rule ever failed you?

Patient: No, it hasn't, except for working. I told my husband it wasn't a good idea for me to work full time because it could cause attacks. But volunteering 2 or 3 days is fine. He agrees. Volunteering gets me out of the house for at least 4 or 5 hours, and I'm around people that I like a lot.

Therapist: Any reason why you settle on 2 or 3 days instead of 1 day or 5 days?

Patient: Well, 2 or 3 days is all the volunteer time they need. Besides, we are planning on moving, and so my husband likes me doing 2 days a week of volunteering, and then the rest of the week I can pack.

Therapist: You're moving?

Patient: Yes, to Oak Lawn. It's a suburb a little bit southwest of where we are living right now. Gets us closer to family. Besides, all our friends around here have moved. My neighbors have moved, and so it's kind of hard on me.

Therapist: Is that going to be a good move for you and your health?

Patient: I hope. But it'll be tough, too. This has been my house for 29 years.

Therapist: It was your family's home?

Patient: Right, it was my mom and dad's, and that was the only house that I've known.

Therapist: And your parents?

Patient: Both are deceased. And I was the only child. So it was kind of hard at first and everything. For my husband, it's the same thing. His mom and dad are deceased, too. And right now he is seeing a doctor and a therapist because he has never really mourned his parents. And I told him, "Now you know how I feel." Because I mourned, but I didn't really mourn. And that really affected me, too.

Therapist: So you have more mourning to do?

Patient: Not really, no. I mean, like some occasions, like on Mother's Day, Father's Day, little things here and there, or anniversaries and birthdays will come up, but it is not so bad. But my husband has never mourned. He just took it real lightly, and myself, I was the other way around.

Therapist: And how long ago was. . . .

Patient: Ah, my dad was 12 years ago, and my mom 11.

Therapist: All right, so they were very close together.

Patient: Um, only 9 weeks between them. So, it was hard. But I had family and friends that were around.

Therapist: All right. And you got through things.

Patient: Yeah, I got through. But then 4 or 5 years ago, these things came up.

Therapist: These attacks started happening.

Patient: Right. Because at first, in 1982, I started getting the attacks. My family doctor said it was epilepsy, and I started taking Dilantin for them.

Therapist: Was the diagnosis made by a neurologist or based on a battery of tests for seizure disorder?

Patient: Not really.

Therapist: What was your response to the Dilantin?

Patient: It seemed to work pretty well at first. But about a year later, the attacks came back, and my doctor sent me to a specialist at an epilepsy clinic.

Therapist: And. . . .

Patient: He said the tests were inconclusive, but because my first attack happened in the presence of another person—my husband—he said I probably did have a grad mal seizure. It may be a mild case of epilepsy, because there had only been a few attacks. He said it may not be a problem if I can avoid stress.

Therapist: That was about 14 years ago. But recently you've had more attacks. What does your current neurologist say?

Patient: He says the tests results are not clear. He thinks that what I'm having now are more like panic attacks, so he sent me to a psychiatrist who gives me medication, and I see a therapist in his office for counseling on reducing anxiety.

Therapist: How do you experience the attacks you've been having lately?

Patient: Oh, I just get like really tense and I stop breathing, but then I tell myself, "Breathe, breathe, just keep breathing." And then it's like I'm lifting weights. That's the way I feel, and then I . . . my arm drops down, and then maybe a few seconds later it will start up again, and I have to either be laying down on a couch or laying on a bed flat so I don't fall anyway because I don't want to hurt myself.

Therapist: About how long would that whole episode last?

Patient: The last one I had lasted practically all day, all day long from like 10:00 in the morning to almost 9:00 at night.

Therapist: When was that, the last one?

Patient: Oh, probably about 2 months ago.

Therapist: When was the first one?

Patient: When was the first one? Oh, that was a few moths before we got married. We were planning our wedding, and there was a lot of stuff on my mind. I really got stressed. And that was when they started happening.

Therapist: Can you describe the very first attack?

Patient: The first one I had, I was in bed, and all of a sudden, I was . . . the pain came up my leg into my arm, and I grabbed the bedpost, and it went over to this side, and I grabbed the bedpost, and I just . . . I didn't know what it was. And I just called my husband. I just called him and called him, and he finally came in. And then I got out of the bed, and then it started again, and I sat on the floor, and I held his hand, and it went the same way and everything. And we didn't know what to do. I mean, we tried calling my doctor to come to the house, and they wanted me to come in, but I couldn't go in.

Therapist: So what were you thinking and feeling when it happened?

Patient: Oh, God, I didn't know what to think. It was like demons coming in.

Therapist: Demons?

Patient: Not really demons, but like a scary roller-coaster ride where you really get scared. And that's how I felt. Kind of like sharp and tight. Tightness. Then moving, like shocks.

Therapist: Tightness and shocks.

Patient:	Yeah, coming all the way up and going down, and then it would start all over again. And I had it like that for 3 or 4 hours.
Therapist:	So these were shooting sensations?
Patient:	Yes.
Therapist:	And what about other things you noticed?
Patient:	Really, those are the only kinds of experiences I get.
Therapist:	Anything such as a change in your breathing?
Patient:	Oh, yes. My heart goes really fast, and then I would stop breathing. Like, I would get scared, and I would. . . .
Therapist:	Hold your breath.
Patient:	Yeah. And then what I was told, to breathe, breathe, continue breathing but slowly. Pace your breathing.
Therapist:	What kind of feelings did you have?
Patient:	Scariness. I was very scared.
Therapist:	How scared?
Patient:	Um, just as scared as you can get. Just wishing they were over.
Therapist:	So scared that you thought something disastrous might happen?
Patient:	No, not really. Not that I was going to die or anything. I was just scared. I was just, I wished they would just get out of my system. I wish I never had them. I wished they would never come back.
Therapist:	Have you ever experienced anything like that in your life before?
Patient:	No, no, that was the first time it's ever happened.
Therapist:	Well, it seems you mentioned something similar that happened when going on a ride.
Patient:	No. It was just so scary. You want it to go away and never come back. But they just do when I get all stressed out.
Therapist:	Do you know anybody else who has had anything like that?
Patient:	Um, not really. Wait, I take that back. I do have a cousin who has panic attacks, but I've never seen him have them. I'm the first one in the family that's ever had seizures.
Therapist:	Can you say a little about your parents and what it was like growing up?

She reports that her mother was emotionally distant, perhaps even to the point of being neglectful. Her father was gone often because of his work, and when he was around, she craved his attention. There was little physical manifestation of love and caring from him, but nevertheless, she spent as much time around him as she could. She had no best friend growing up, and she finished only 3 years of high school before she got married to Fred, who is 7 years older than she. I learned that whenever she was sick, her mother made her go to school anyway. This became a point of contention among her parents. When her father was home, he made sure she was seen by their family physician. I then asked about her parents' health.

> *Therapist:* So it sounds like while you had some illness when you were growing up, your parents were for the most part quite healthy.
>
> *Patient:* Yeah, they were fine up until their deaths and everything like that, and fine.
>
> *Therapist:* But their deaths were not really a surprise. Weren't they both quite ill?
>
> *Patient:* Yes. Both of them had cancer. Yeah. But it was hard.
>
> *Therapist:* Did you have any particular kind of reaction around the time of their deaths?
>
> *Patient:* Well, I remember when they operated on my dad the second time. And they found the cancer, and the doctor did not come into the room, but he called my mother to say that may dad had cancer. It was in between the liver and pancreas, and it was inoperable and all, and when my mother told me, I just screamed and said, "I hate God. I just hate him," and my mother took me to the side and she said, "Don't you ever say that." You know, I was just so mad. You just get mad. Anything just comes out of your mouth. And the same thing when my mother was ill. My aunt would bring her to the doctor, and I'd be talking to her on the phone, but it would be going in one ear and out the other. You just didn't want to hear it. It was just, you know, I didn't want to hear about it at all.

It is clear that Kathleen has strong and mixed feelings about doctors. On the one hand, she appears to look up to them as father figures, but on the other hand, she can be very angry with them when they cannot fix things or, for that matter, when they do not discuss painful news face to face but rather call to relay bad news.

> *Therapist:* So you couldn't hear it, you couldn't tolerate it. . . .
>
> *Patient:* No.
>
> *Therapist:* But you were also very angry.

Patient: Yeah, I was very angry, because I wish I could go back a few times and say like where are important papers that I need? You know, just have a talk with them. That'll be the first thing I do when I get up there. I'm going to say to God, "Why? Why did you take them?" But then I think that God did not want me to watch them suffer or to have to take care of them if they got worse. So I think that they were taken from me when they were just beginning to get sick. I probably didn't really want to take care of them. Ah, it hurt, but in the other sense, I think it was much better.

A sense of comfort seeking and entitlement are present. It appears that she avoids difficult situations and finds it easier to externalize.

Therapist: Because it could have been worse, for them and for you.

Patient: Correct.

In the following discussion, I endeavor to elicit her explanatory model of her illness. Although she initially denies having any explanation, gentle prompting helps to articulate it.

Therapist: What do you suppose is the reason you get these attacks?

Patient: I really wish I could answer that question. I don't know. I don't know at all.

Therapist: Now, I know you're not a doctor.

Patient: No.

Therapist: But I also know that most people try to make sense of things that happen in their life, and they think about the different kinds of explanations, and sometimes those explanations help them to sort things out and to sort of put things to rest. What kind of thoughts have you had about that?

Patient: I just wish they would leave me and just leave me alone. Sometimes I look at some friends and they are all healthy and all, and I say to myself, "Why can't I be like them?" You know, no illnesses or anything, but they could probably have some illnesses that they've never said to me.

Therapist: Well, you said that you wish they would leave. "They" being. . . .

Patient: Meaning either the panic attacks or the epilepsy. I just wish I never had anything. I mean, I don't mind having an occasional cold here and there, but I just wish I could get rid of the attacks.

It may well be that she is externalizing the cause of her illness to others whom she wishes would just leave her alone. Knowing that superstition is not uncommon among families who are Irish immigrants with limited edu-

cation, I make a mental note of it rather than pursue it at the risk of ruptur-
ing a still developing therapeutic alliance.

Therapist: Before, you said you'd really be satisfied if you just had a definite
              answer to the question "Is it panic or epilepsy or both?" Then
              you said your life would be. . . .

Patient: I'd be fine. I'd be happy.

Therapist: That sounds like two different things. In one instance, you're
              willing to settle for just an answer, and in the other one, you say
              you want it to go away.

Patient: Well, I would like to just lead a normal life, have no illnesses,
              no nothing.

Therapist: Do you know anybody who leads that kind of life?

Patient: No. I mean I know a lot of people, they have illnesses and back-
              aches and this, that, and the other, but nobody's perfect.

Therapist: Well, what about yourself?

Patient: No. I'm not perfect.

Therapist: Well, so then you would expect that you wouldn't have perfect
              health then.

Patient: No. But I just wish that I never came across having these, but
              somebody must have wanted me to have them.

Therapist: Somebody?

Patient: Somebody. I don't know who, but they chose me.

Therapist: Sort of like a spell?

Patient: Well, not a spell, but I've seen people that have gone into my
              neurologist's office, and they are worse off than me. I mean there
              was a little boy that was in a wheelchair, and I mean I said to
              myself, "My god, that could be me. That could have been me. I
              could have been in a wheelchair, couldn't walk or talk or drive
              or anything or walk, or you know, my head could be in a brace
              of something like that or, I'm lucky. I'm lucky I can hold a job,
              walk, go to concerts, and lead a normal life."

Again, the sense of externalization appears to be a key aspect of her explanatory model.

Therapist: So maybe things aren't so bad after all.

Patient: No, they're not. They're not.

Therapist: What's your expectation about your condition and your life over
              the next 6 months?

I asked this rather standard question to elicit her level of readiness for change, but she appears to interpret the question quite differently and concretely.

Patient: Well, hopefully to get out of our house. Moved into a new either home or apartment or whatever. And, hopefully, we will start having a family. And just be happy as pie.

Therapist: All right. How does the idea of starting a family sound for you?

Patient: Sounds good. I'd like to.

Therapist: Any reservations about it?

Patient: No. I was an only child and I didn't like it. I'd like to have at least two children if possible, so at least they have somebody to hang onto, and I just don't want it to be my husband and myself when we get old. I'd like to have grandchildren and all. Something to look forward to.

Therapist: When you say that, your eyes shifted one direction and then the other. It's almost as if your words said one thing and your body was saying something else.

This is my first inkling that the prospect of having and raising children is one of considerable ambivalence to her.

Patient: No. I didn't know that.

Therapist: Yeah.

Patient: But I'm looking forward to getting everything together.

Therapist: Sometimes people can be looking forward to something a lot but still have misgivings. Do you have that experience sometimes?

Patient: No, no, I don't have any misgivings. I just want to have a nice life with my husband, raise a nice family, and just get on with life. Be nice and happy. We have occasional problems in the family. Everybody will have problems like that, and just grow old together. That's what I think.

Therapist: What's the likelihood that this is going to happen?

Patient: I think it will happen.

Therapist: Even with all these uncertain medical concerns?

Patient: I think it will. I really want to get down to it to figure out what the heck is wrong with me.

Therapist: There's going to be three possible answers. One is that it's something that is very well defined but which may or may not be treatable. A second possibility is that there really isn't anything at all that medical tests can pick up, at least at this stage of the illness. And third is that it might be something that can be diagnosed, but because of attitudes and beliefs that you have, it may get worse. If you could get that answer today and be absolutely certain that that was the exact diagnosis and it wasn't anything else—it was going to be one of those three—which of those three would you find easiest to live with? Which would you find most difficult to live with?

I pose what has been called The Questions (Dreikurs, 1967) or its variant, The Miracle Question, and she has considerable difficulty dealing with it.

Patient: I would just want to be happy. Just be very happy.

Therapist: But you only have those three choices.

Patient: I couldn't answer you right now. I don't know.

Therapist: You don't.

Patient: No. Not right now.

Therapist: What's keeping you from knowing right now?

Patient: I really don't know offhand.

Therapist: Well, let's say you don't know now with absolute certainty. What inklings do you have?

Patient: Like of . . . ?

Therapist: Well, which of those three would be the most difficult for you to accept? Just based on what you know about yourself as a person and how your life has gone.

Patient: I really don't know offhand.

Therapist: Let me ask you something else.

Patient: Sure.

Therapist: Could you demonstrate what that tightness was like, without describing? Could you just show me in your body what it was like?

Patient: Sure. It would be, it would come up my leg, be real tight.

Therapist: Without words.

Patient: Okay. Come up here, up to my. . . .

Therapist: But you can't use words.

Patient: Real tight. Go across, down, and down.

Therapist: If I were to come into that room where you and your husband were that day of your first attack, what would I see?

Patient: He would probably be sitting up against the couch on the floor, and I would have a hold of both of his hands because at that time I was afraid if somebody would let go of my hands that I was going to fall or anything like that. I was on the floor, but still I had to hold onto somebody's hands, or if they even just tried to let go a little bit to get blood back in their fingers, I would feel like I was falling.

Therapist: And if you fell, what's the worst thing that would happen to you?

Patient: Well, I'd fall, I'd fall. I'd get back up. I've fallen quite a few times. I fell in the shower two times. When I feel an attack coming on, I get down on the floor. And the next thing I know is that I have rug burns on my nose.

Therapist: What's the worst thing that could happen to you?

Patient: Well, I couldn't die from these.

Therapist: You're sure of that?

Patient: Yeah. My husband always tells me, but I think it's in anger, that he says he would leave me. Because he is just tired of these. But I think he just says it because he's mad, because these keep coming on, and on, and on. But I just get these, I think, when I'm all stressed out, when I have two or three different things on my mind at the one time. And I just get so stressed that I just go into having the attacks.

Therapist: And you said he was very angry with you?

Patient: Yeah, he gets mad, but then he goes out to cool off. He takes a ride or whatever, and it doesn't bother me.

Therapist: It doesn't bother you that he is angry at you?

Patient: Well, I understand now because we have been through it so many times over the years. He just goes off and just drives around, and then he will come back, because he says he can't stay around because he knows how it will be. He comes back and then he's okay. He understands.

Therapist: What does he understand?

Patient: Well, he understands that I'm going through these things and he wants me to get better. He does. Because he wants both of us to have children and carry on a normal good life.

Therapist: Have you had any couple counseling?

Patient: No. No. Not at all.

Therapist: But right now you're getting some individual counseling for yourself.

Patient: And he's getting counseling himself because he has not gotten over his grief with his parents. So he likes going to that, too.

Therapist: Is it possible there may be some relationship issues involved here?

Patient: I mean, if we ever had to go to a marriage counselor, we'd go, but you know, I mean I don't think we would say no to it. We'd go and just see if it was that or if it was both of our, I mean my, panic attacks and his grief just to see. I'd do that. I'd be game.

Therapist: What is the earliest experience you can remember as a child?

The purpose here is to elicit some confirmation for my developing clinical formulation through the use of the projective technique of early recollections.

Patient: Earliest thing. Hmm. I remember getting in trouble with my dad. My girl friend in the neighborhood and I went across the street and were playing like in a new home they were building. Both our fathers found our little tricycles at the corner, but not us. So they found us in the new house, and oh boy, did we get a whipping.

Therapist: How old were you at the time?

Patient: I was about 4 and she was about 3, so.

Therapist: And whose idea was it?

Patient: Well, we got up to the corner, and our other neighbors were across playing in there, and we just kind of looked at each other and said, "Let's go for it."

Therapist: Which part of that whole experience do you remember most vividly?

Patient: The spanking. It hurt.

Therapist: How were you spanked?

Patient: We were standing up. Both the dads had to carry the bikes back. Then they spanked us and told us not to go over there anymore.

Therapist: How about another early memory?

Patient: There was another time when I went into a swimming pool at a neighbor's house two doors down. I kept asking my mom, "I'm going swimming." "No you're not. No you're not." I said, "I'm going swimming." So I went into the pool, and we were up to our chins in the water, and my dad found out that I was in the pool, and so did the other neighbor, it was the same girl, oh boy. We got hit coming out of the pool.

Therapist: What part of that do you remember most vividly?

Patient:	Um, that the water was up to my chin and I could barely breathe.
Therapist:	What was your feeling with water being up to your chin and barely being able to breathe?
Patient:	Nothing. My neighbor was asking if I was supposed to be in that pool, and I said no.
Therapist:	What's your recollection about that?
Patient:	Well, just being in the pool and having fun.
Therapist:	And how were you feeling?
Patient:	Fine. I was feeling fine.
Therapist:	Was it an adventure? Was it scary?
Patient:	No, it wasn't scary. No, it was fun. I like to swim.
Therapist:	All right. But you said you were concerned whether you were going to be able to breathe like that.
Patient:	Well, a little bit scared. Because I was on my tippy toes with the water up to my chin because it was a 4-foot pool, and I was under that height.
Therapist:	Sure. And how old were you at the time?
Patient:	Um, 4.

These two recollections suggest that Kathleen engages in adventurous and daring behavior that she knows is unacceptable—to her parents—but results in her receiving attention in the form of a spanking from her father. She gets the physical attention and "caring" she so craves, presumably because she cannot easily get it in ways other than through a spanking. Because memories of the past are constructions that reflect a person's reality in the present, it is assumed that themes and pattern of these recollections are operative in her current personality dynamics and behavior.

Therapist:	It sounds like you did some pretty daring things as a child, and that you were very independent, too.
Patient:	Yes and no.
Therapist:	Well how about the "no" part? In what way were you not daring and independent?
Patient:	This was really stupid when I look back at it. My parents used to go to a neighbor's house on Saturday night, and I could not fall asleep until my mother was back in the house. And I could never understand it until now.
Therapist:	And what's your understanding now?

Patient: Well, now I think that I just had to have her in the house to feel safe. That she had to be in the house before I could fall asleep. And when I got older and used to be out late at night, she wouldn't fall asleep until I got home.

It appears that she needs her mother in a different way: proximity, but not necessarily the closeness of a caring touch.

Therapist: And somehow she understood that, and accepted that, and your life went on and her life went on.

Patient: Yes.

Therapist: If we put your husband in your mother's place, would he have understood that?

Patient: Yes, he would. He'd understand.

Therapist: And he wouldn't have gotten mad at you?

Patient: No. See, I was always afraid when I was growing up that when I would get married I'd be afraid if my husband would go out for the night that I wouldn't be able to fall asleep until he got home. But it's actually the other way around. I could fall asleep, and then he would come in. So we have made a pact. I told him that if he spends the night at a friend's house, he should call me. And if he forgets, I let him know.

Therapist: How do you let him know?

Patient: Oh, I give him a few nice words. I'll have an argument with him, and he says, "Okay, yeah, I know. I'm dumb. I know I did a dumb thing." But we've got a good understanding. A good friendship and marriage.

Therapist: Who are you most like, your mother or your father?

Patient: I'm a lot like my dad. And I'm like my mom in some ways, too. But more like my dad.

Therapist: Which one spoiled you more than the other?

Patient: My dad. Oh god, my dad. I always went a lot of places with him. To the store. He'd say, "Hey, let's go to the store." I'd get in the car and go with him. But I was close to my mom in a different way. But when my dad died, it really hit me. Probably because he was the first person I was very close to that died. To this day, I don't know that answer, but I think that's what it is.

In the following discussion, I first try to universalize her experience and then offer an indirect hypnotic suggestion.

Therapist: That makes sense. [*Pause*] How you've described your symptoms is not much different than the way other people who have your symptoms describe them. Oftentimes they tell similar kinds of early life experiences as you've described. And very often, there is a sense of where they are doing one of two things. They are either holding on really tight to themselves or feeling like their breath is holding them in very, very tight. And you want to know what tends to happen with those individuals? After a period of time, something very interesting happens. And they wouldn't have predicted it. Other people they know never would have guessed that it would have happened, but it happens. You know what it is?

Patient: No.

Therapist: All of a sudden, out of the clear blue, that sense of tightness starts easing up. It tightens up a little bit, eases up a little bit, and then it is gone.

Patient: That's very good.

Therapist: And that means then that your breathing kind of starts back into a normal rhythm again because breath is something that we don't have to even think about. There is an automaticity to it. It just happens. It's like your heart, and when the breathing comes back, it's as if their concerns and their problems may still be there, but they don't seem to be quite the same. There is a slightly different coloring to them. The texture of those concerns is a little bit different. Many of the things in their lives that were going well before continue to go well. And some of the other things in their life that weren't going quite so well really start becoming less of a problem. Now, that doesn't mean they are perfect anymore and not that everything has gone away, but there is not quite that sense of impending concern. And do you know why I'm thinking that's going to happen?

Patient: No.

In the following discussion, I begin offering an extended interpretation and a reframing of her condition and attacks—through her early recollections—as they relate to her needs and her father's response.

Therapist: The story you told about the bicycles and the new house and about the swimming pool, both of those situations in the short run didn't seem like they were absolutely happy endings. But your life went on after that.

Patient: Yeah, it did.

Therapist: And it was that little point in time, seconds, maybe a couple of minutes, and you got past the spanking. It came from the individual who was probably the closest person in your life.

Patient: And they were just trying to teach us.

Therapist:	Yes.
Patient:	Not to do wrong.
Therapist:	Yes. And they may have been trying to teach you something else, too. Probably even more so, and that is how to stay alive, to stay healthy. I think that's what the lesson was in both of those stories.
Patient:	I think so, too.
Therapist:	And that's a legacy that your parents gave to you. You'll always have those memories. Things weren't going well for a while. They were very exciting up until that time when you were running around the house and in the pool, and then this little bit of reality comes in, but nothing really bad happens. You don't die; you don't lose privileges or get grounded for 10 years. But out of that experience, something good came. Your relationship was restored with your father. I'm sure he loved you as much as you did.
Patient:	Oh, god yeah. Yes, he did.
Therapist:	And I'm wondering if that pattern, that little pattern, may repeat itself just ever so occasionally in your life in a little miniature fashion.
Patient:	It might. I think it does. Because I miss my dad a lot. I really miss him. I wish he could be here when we have children. He would miss them.
Therapist:	And here's what I am going to suggest to you, Kathleen. That one of the ways that you have been able to keep that fond memory of your father alive happens in your relationship with your husband.
Patient:	Right.
Therapist:	Okay, so you two mix it up a little bit, but what is it that ends up coming out of that? He shows you are still together. You've got a life plan. It's maybe a little. . . .
Patient:	Rocky here and there.
Therapist:	Yes. And the future may not be absolutely clear. You're discussing having children and growing old together and having grandchildren, but you never know exactly how every step will be.
Patient:	We're just going to have to go day by day.
Therapist:	Right. And, you have a unique way of remembering your father, and I think the important part of this whole thing is the experience you have of feeling energized and so alive that is happen-

ing in both instances. When you were a little girl and even with the tightening up, there is a sense of aliveness that's there because it's not like the rest of your everyday life experiences. And you're in a very interesting situation: As you change that little pattern that you have with your husband, you'll be changing your relationship, your relationship with your father. There will likely be a new place for him in your life and in your heart.

Patient: What do you mean?

Therapist: It may be that at some point in time that inner sense that something isn't right will start going away. As it goes away, you won't need to remember your father through the experience of breathlessness, tightening sensations, and symptoms that way you did in the past. Instead, you will be able to remember him without having the symptoms. You'll still be able to love him, cherish him, and remember him. And, it means that your life will be able to go on and be fine, and your life with your husband is going to go on without much need for the symptoms. So that's what I think might happen. But you know what? It might take a different tack. But you're going to be the one that will know that.

Here, I'm scripting a new story, an alternative explanatory model for her symptoms and her need for them, by recasting the relationship between needing the support of her father—and other father figures—and the breath cycle that brings on her attacks. The implication is that she can get attention and caring from significant others without having to experience dramatic symptoms and put up with the side effects of medications she might not need to take. Apparently, this makes some sense to Kathleen, as she responds affirmatively both verbally and nonverbally.

Patient: [*Nodding affirmatively*] Yeah.

Therapist: Okay.

Patient: That's right.

The session concludes with a discussion of a disposition plan.

REVIEW OF THE COMPREHENSIVE ASSESSMENT

The assessment consultation was completed in this 90-minute face-to-face session. Brief phone discussions were held with the referring neurologist, psychiatrist, and therapist. The neurologist was convinced that Kathleen's diagnosis was psychogenic seizures, and he would not accede to her request for Dilantin. The psychiatrist indicated that although Kathleen claimed that Paxil was helping, she also reported side effects, including decreased libido

TABLE 8.1
Summary of Comprehensive Assessment of the Case of Kathleen

Assessment factor	Minimum responsiveness
Level of illness progression and impact	Appears to be situationally disabling
Illness representation or explanatory model	External, negative
Adequacy of health behaviors and exposure Hx	Poor; high: secondhand cigarette smoke
Early parental bond and ACE (abuse or neglect)	Insecure; severe: emotional and sexual
Personal schemas and family narratives	Disability prone
Personality style or disorder	Disorder: borderline, histrionic
Family competence and style	Severely dysfunctional
Religious and spiritual beliefs	Negative and complicating
Patient resources, especially self-capacities	Limited, negative; underdeveloped
Readiness for treatment or capacity for self-mgmt	Low
Adequacy of Tx relationship with other providers	Poor
Alignment of explanatory model and treatment goals	Low
Phase of illness	Looping between Phases 1 and 2

Note. Hx = history; ACE = adverse childhood experience; self-mgmt = self-management; Tx = treatment.

and sexual performance. Furthermore, he was not convinced that she had an Axis I disorder that was responsive to medications. He wanted to discontinue the medication but anticipated that this would meet with considerable opposition from her. The therapist was frustrated in efforts to engage her in any behavioral techniques to reduce stress and indicated that she did not seem to comprehend the therapist's questions and instructions. All three providers were frustrated with her, and they implied that they would be more than happy to have me work with her exclusively.

Some key points of the evaluation are noted here, and the rest are summarized in Table 8.1. Prior to the assessment and according to her current providers, it appeared that Kathleen's level of illness progression was mild to moderate, but its impact appeared to be moderately disabling. However, on the basis of my assessment and interaction with her, it is only situationally disabling.

Her explanatory model is quite interesting in that it is externalized (i.e., her symptoms are caused by outside forces) and that it is a double disorder—that is, a panic disorder superimposed on a generalized seizure disorder. She appears to have no insight into the intrapersonal or interpersonal determinants of her condition. Her attachment style seems to be insecure, probably reflecting the extensive neglect she experienced at the hands of her mother. It is noteworthy that she was denied caring, concern, and even medical help when she was ill as a child by her mother, but received just the opposite by her father. Her personal resources seem quite limited, and her self-capacities, particularly for self-soothing, appear to be undeveloped. She would probably merit the diagnosis of personality disorder NOS characterized by borderline, histrionic, and passive–aggressive features. Kathleen appears to be "looping" between Phases 1 and 2 of her illness, in that she shifts back and forth between crisis and stabilization (Fennell, 2003). I am hopeful that focused psychotherapeutic strategies directed at her illness denial that feeds this looping and blocks her from moving to Phase 3 will be effective. Finally, based on the results of my comprehensive assessment, my clinical impression is that the presentation she describes is more consistent with psychogenic seizures, also called psuedoseizures. As mentioned previously, psychogenic seizures can be diagnosed in individuals who had previously met the criteria for a seizure disorder or never met those criteria.

CASE CONCEPTUALIZATION—PATTERN ANALYSIS

The referring physician's basic concern was Kathleen's apparent treatment resistance and insistence that she be prescribed antiepileptic medications even though she does not meet the criteria for a focal or generalized seizure disorder. The following pattern analysis provides a means of understanding her reported "treatment resistance" and suggests strategies that might be effective in working with her.

Precipitants

Kathleen experiences boredom, sensations of emptiness, and feelings of being unloved (psychological). Usually, these arise after the experiences of loss, demands from her husband, or other's expectations that she begin a family, get a job, and so on (social). Faced with this sense of emptiness, actual or perceived loss, and demands—particularly relational demands—Kathleen engages in rumination. Left unchecked, her ruminations—that is, distractions such as her volunteer job—build and result in hyperventilation and breathlessness (biological). In the past, she has faced several stressors, including her marriage in 1982, her parents dying 4 to 5 years later, her husband's graduation from college, and recent discussions about starting a family. The prospect of childbearing appears to be fraught with several concerns for her, such as whether she is healthy enough to be a mother, whether it requires that she stop her anxiolytic medication, whether the relationship can accommodate a child, and so on. She reports major attacks prior to her marriage, at the time her husband was graduating from college, and recently with discussions of beginning a family.

Presentation

Breathlessness leads to a sensation of increasing tightness, which leads to experiencing attacks (biological). When others respond to her symptoms—particularly her husband, physicians, or other male health care providers—she experiences the comforting touch of a father figure. They are mobilized by her distress and provide her attention, physical support, caring, or concern, even though it appears to involve a noxious element, that is, spanking by father, medication side effects, and so on (social). As a result, Kathleen experiences a sensation of aliveness, self-worth, and validation as a loved and cared-for person (psychological).

Predisposition

A unique set of predisposing factors appears to be operative. Particularly noteworthy is her style of knowing and processing reality. It is a somatizing style in which, instead of experiencing distress as affects, such as fear or despair, she "converts" them into unpleasant physical sensations or medical symptoms. Often concurrent with this style is alexithymia, that is, the inability to experience and label feelings that are the coin of the realm in the therapeutic process (biological). Her schemas include excitement seeking, entitlement, comfort seeking, and the need to be in control at all costs. As a child, Kathleen seemed to crave her father's attention and closeness and would engage in daring and "disobedient" behaviors to get it, even if it resulted in a spanking. Later, she sought excitement to demonstrate her independence and worthwhileness, getting attention from father figures, such as her husband and health care providers (psychological). Her family values include obedience, stoicism, independence, and physical discipline. Her family narrative is something like the following: "People should be responsive to others' misfortune and pain, and discipline means caring" (social). Because of her somatizing style, she has a limited capacity for understanding and verbalizing her needs. Accordingly, she explains and attributes her symptoms and chronic illness to external influences, that is, demons and others (explanatory model). Given her cultural roots, that is, first-generation Irish with limited education, such an attribution is not unreasonable.

Perpetuants

To the extent to which she experiences pain, attacks, and even medication side effects, and the concomitant attention and efforts of her husband and health care providers, Kathleen achieves the sense of caring and control that she needs and demands.

In short, Kathleen's reported treatment resistance can be understood in terms of her somatizing style and her need to be in control and get her way.

Somatizing individuals like Kathleen can be particularly challenging for medical personnel and psychotherapists who find it easier to work with patients who can identify and label feelings and pain sensations with some degree of preciseness and coherence. Unfortunately, those with a somatizing style tend to be more concrete and less coherent and precise, and appear to be uncooperative. Working effectively with such patients requires a different approach on the part of the health care provider. Table 8.2 summarizes this pattern analysis.

TREATMENT ISSUES AND STRATEGY

Based on the pattern analysis, the following treatment focus is suggested; Table 8.2 summarizes these interventions and their potential sequencing. Note that the numbering represents the order in which interventions are sequenced; that is, coaching is first, whereas schema work, re-storying, explanatory model, and family narrative are second, followed by coaching on controlled breathing.

Given that Kathleen's biopsychosocial triggers are relatively circumscribed, the initial therapeutic focus probably should be on coaching her to keep herself busy with her volunteer work and other activities that can reduce the likelihood of rumination. The goal is to limit the likelihood that the conditions that can lead to an "attack" will be activated [Intervention/Sequence 1].

Next, treatment would include some additional individual sessions with Kathleen to deal with her schemas, family narrative, and relationship with her husband. This work would build on the initial therapeutic efforts in the assessment consultation, particularly with refocusing and reframing her relationship with her father such that she can recall and reexperience his caring and concern without activating her "attack" cycle [Intervention/Sequence 2].

Finally, coaching in the guise of health-focused counseling strategies that teach her to control and monitor her breathing and other stress-management techniques could be used [Intervention/Sequence 3]. It is quite likely that the therapist failed in her efforts to help Kathleen master these skills, because to acquire and use such techniques would mean that Kathleen could not reexperience her connection with her father.

TREATMENT PROCESS AND OUTCOME OF THE CASE

A follow-up appointment was made with me, and work began on the focal issues previously described. We met 2 weeks later for another session. After that, her husband participated in a session. During that time, Kathleen was weaned off Paxil and terminated treatment with the psychiatrist and

TABLE 8.2
Pattern Analysis and Treatment Strategy for the Case of Kathleen

Pattern factor	Formulation/treatment target	Intervention/sequence
Precipitating factor	(P) Bored, unloved, and empty sensations; (S) Losses, relational demands, family expectations; (B) Rumination breathlessness	1. Coaching—keep busy and other rumination-reduction techniques
Predisposing factor	(B) Somatizing style, alexithymia; (P) Excitement seeking, entitlement, and control; (S) Family values of obedience and "discipline means caring"	2. Schema work 2. Revise explanatory model 2. Re-story family narrative
Presentation response	(B) "Attack" or touch of father figure; (P) Sense of aliveness; (S) Mobilization of physical support, caring, concern	3. Coaching—controlled breathing and stress-management techniques
Perpetuating factor	(B/P/S) Experiencing attacks/pain achieves caring and control	2. Schema/explanatory model work 2. Re-story family narrative

Note. Letters in parentheses represent biological (B), psychological (P), and sociological (S) factors.

therapist doing stress-management work. She did want to continue with the neurologist and negotiated follow-up appointments at 4-month intervals. In a brief phone consultation with the neurologist, it was agreed that "stress-induced attacks" was an acceptable diagnosis to everyone—Kathleen, the neurologist, and me. In our sessions, she agreed that keeping busy enough and not ruminating was essential. She continued to be amenable to reframing and re-storying in which she could cherish the memory without having to get sick, without it triggering attacks, or without needing to take medication with significant side effects. It was clear that there remained relationship issues between Kathleen and her husband, and we scheduled additional sessions focused on these. It has been 6 months since our last appointment, and Kathleen reports that there have been no attacks. In our conjoint sessions, the couple decided that childbearing was probably not wise at this time, and instead they decided to check into adopting an older child. This decision relieved considerable angst for Kathleen regarding the possibility that she might neglect the infant or young child, as her mother had done to her. Given that the application process might take up to 18 months, the couple felt comfortable with having sufficient time in which to prepare for this event. They also became involved in a support group of parents who are planning for adoption.

CONCLUDING NOTE

This case illustrates the process of approaching, assessing, and initially working with patients with chronic illness who have been labeled by other health care providers as "difficult" or "treatment resistant." With Kathleen, the nature of her "resistance" was in part a function of her somatizing style. Clinicians who understand and can accommodate this style are often able to engage otherwise challenging patients like Kathleen in the treatment process. Another part of her resistance was her externalizing explanatory model with dynamics that confounded her illness and her relationship with her father and other father figures. As this was sorted out and processed, Kathleen became more able to take responsibility for changes in her life.

9

COUNSELING STRATEGIES
IN CHRONIC ILLNESS

This chapter highlights the use of health-focused counseling strategies with chronic physical illness. As noted earlier, health-focused counseling strategies are the mainstay of treatment and are particularly appropriate for patients in which health-focused counseling rather than health-focused psychotherapy is indicated. Patients who are particularly well suited for health-focused counseling are those who are receptive to treatment advice and skill training and for whom treatment of their chronic illness is not impeded by illness or by significant psychological factors—that is, a personality or substance use disorder—undermine or compromise treatment compliance. Often, these individuals have received some form of health counseling or patient education from medical or other health care providers but may not have responded fully because the advice or other interventions were not tailored to their psychological dynamics and contextual dynamics.

As in the previously cases (that is, those described in chaps. 7 and 8), an extended evaluation session was arranged with the patient, with the understanding that, if indicated and if there was mutual agreement, additional sessions might be scheduled. The following case demonstrates the use of health counseling strategies with an individual who, despite conscientious adherence to a self-management program for her chronic sinusitis, has experienced a worsening of her condition. Surgery has been recommended, but she wants a second opinion on nonsurgical options, including psychotherapy, that might make a difference.

BACKGROUND OF THE CASE

Ellen is a 47-year-old married Caucasian woman who is seeking an alternative to surgery for her worsening chronic sinusitis condition. She was referred by a friend for whom I had provided health-focused psychotherapy in the past. This friend had told her I had offered her suggestions that helped her avoid sinus surgery. Ellen called for an appointment, hoping that I would offer her therapy or some different treatment recommendations. She had experienced respiratory problems, particularly sinusitis and allergic rhinitis, since adolescence, but her symptoms had worsened considerably over the past year. Particularly bothersome was postnasal drip that led to choking and disturbed sleep and sinus headaches that were increasing in number and intensity. She had undergone several courses of antibiotic therapy during the past year, but her chronic sinusitis and allergic rhinitis continued to worsen, and surgery was being considered. She sought this consultation in the hope that there might be additional treatment and self-management options that could make a difference and eliminate the need for surgery, which she considered a last resort. Ellen was married and had one grandchild and two adolescent sons living at home with her and her husband. She had worked as a hairstylist for approximately 8 years.

SESSION TRANSCRIPTION

Following are segments of the transcription—along with commentary—of a 90-minute initial consultation session with Ellen. During the course of this consultation, I had two objectives: (a) to complete a relatively comprehensive biopsychosocial assessment of her experience of her chronic illness and life and, on the basis of this assessment, (b) to ascertain the extent to which health counseling or psychotherapeutic strategies might be indicated and her amenability to such interventions. After introductions, the session begins:

Therapist: Could you describe the symptoms associated with your chronic sinusitis, particularly the one which you are experiencing now?

Patient: They start with minor symptoms like postnasal drip and a sore throat, then proceed to throat swelling, which makes me feel like I'm choking. This is especially bad at night and on awakening. Then it leads to a buildup of pressure and blockage in my ears, which usually leads to a sinus infection and a sinus headache. Other symptoms include fatigue and nausea. I have most of these symptoms daily. They don't seem to ever stop, and so over the years, I've gotten used to them.

Therapist: You mentioned four specific symptoms; which is the most problematic for you?

Patient: If you asked me today, it would be headaches. Other times, it's the postnasal drip and choking. Sometimes it's the fatigue from fighting infections all the time. The sore throat is there all the time.

Therapist: How often do you have infections? How many times a year?

Patient: This last one has gone on for most of the year. In the past, I have had episodes that have lasted a few months two or three times a year. But this year it has gone on and on and on for months now. I just finished my fifth course of antibiotics.

Therapist: What antibiotics have been prescribed?

Patient: I think I've had all of them. The last two have been Bactrim and Augmentin.

Therapist: How many years have you been experiencing sinus symptoms?

Patient: A long, long time. Probably since I was 7 years old. It wasn't diagnosed as sinusitis then but usually as strep throat or an ear infection.

Therapist: So this illness has been going on for several years, and you've been experiencing four fairly well defined symptoms. If you put these symptoms together and rate to them on a 1 to 10 scale, with 1 being *very mild* and 10 being *very severe*, what number would you give them right now?

Patient: When I just got this last course of antibiotics, I would say it was 7. But in the last week the symptoms are escalating, and I would say it is to 8 or 9. I'm ready to find another doctor because I'm not really getting better.

Therapist: I hear your frustration with your illness and your treatment. . . . How would you rate your symptoms overall 1 year ago, the best you felt?

Patient: Probably a 3.

Therapist: Has it ever been lower than a 3?

Patient: Probably not.

Therapist: Even as a child?

Patient: No, even then I thought there was something wrong, that I just wasn't feeling as good as my brothers or sisters or friends. I always carried Kleenex around with me. It seemed like I always had sniffles or itchy eyes or itchy nose.

Therapist: In terms of daily functioning, does this illness affect your daily roles and functioning?

Patient: At its worst time, when I am as inflamed as I am right now, definitely yes.

Therapist: What kind of roles and responsibilities are most affected?

Patient: Well, I am a mother and grandmother, and I run a household with my husband. And I have a job. Our son is 14 years old, going on 15, and I spend a lot of time driving him around, all duties a mother of an adolescent is expected to do in suburbia.

Therapist: Looking at your life and your roles and responsibilities, how would you rate your level of functioning or impairment on a scale that runs from 1 to 10, with 1 being *very good functioning and no impairment* and 10 being *very low functioning* and a high level of impairment? How would you rate yourself on that scale when your health is reasonably good?

Patient: Oh, probably a 1.

Therapist: How you would you rate it during the worst period of time in the past 6 months?

Patient: Uhm. I would say around a 7.

Therapist: A 7 is what you rated your symptoms. Are you implying that the intensity of your symptoms affects your functioning to a significant degree?

Patient: Sure. The symptoms affect everything, including my mood and morale. I'm in a mental fog during those times and just getting by.

Therapist: Specifically, how does it affect your functioning at home and on the job?

Patient: I'm able to get out of bed on those days, but I'm not at my best by a long shot. I can usually go to work on those days, but I am crankier and I'm not fun to be around. With all the fluid in my ears, I'm not sure I'm really hearing everything people are telling me. And the headaches, well, they make things even more difficult.

Therapist: I follow you. [*Pause*] How do you understand your illness? How is it that you have this chronic sinus condition?

Patient: My illness is because my sinuses are vulnerable and damaged. And there are environmental conditions that make things worse, such as air pollution. Also, the environment interacts with a person's health status and physiology. Environment is really important in this disease. So, for example, I'm a hairstylist, and the chemicals I use and am exposed to probably affect me. Another factor in this disease is diet. Dairy foods seem to make a big difference. About a year ago I stopped using all milk products, and I felt a lot better, and there was a lot less mucous and postnasal drip than before. I was hoping that this diet change would get rid of the illness, but it didn't. An unrealistic hope, I know. [*Smiles and laughs*]

This initial description of her illness representation and explanatory model suggests that it is medically accurate and realistic and that she has assumed responsibility for her role in managing its treatment.

Therapist: Besides the diet modification, what makes and has made your condition better?

Patient: There are a few things that have been recommended that seemed to help. One is nasal irrigation. Another is that I use steam inhalation to unblock the sinuses.

Therapist: Have either of those made a difference?

Patient: They do make a difference in opening up the sinuses and relieving pressure in the ears, and I use them regularly now.

Therapist: What makes things worse?

Patient: I would say the diet. Some foods produce mucus, which makes everything else worse. So I try to avoid those foods.

Therapist: Before, you mentioned that the environment has an effect. Let's be more specific. What about air quality?

Patient: I notice that air pollution makes a difference. When I'm in industrial areas, my lungs start tightening up. I don't smoke, but when there is smoke around me, I've learned to get out of those areas because it bothers me a lot.

Therapist: What happens when you're exposed to secondhand smoke?

Patient: My sinuses start running and my eyes begin to itch.

Therapist: When it comes to your family and friends, what impact, if any, does your illness have on them?

Patient: Well, my husband is very supportive of me. He understands my suffering and is very helpful. He helps cook healthful foods. He reads food labels and helps me avoid environmental triggers for my respiratory condition. Now, the children, they're another matter. Right now they think the diet thing is a joke for me. They can't seem to understand how something like a dairy product can trigger a sinus headache. But I've only been making diet changes in the past year, so they'll get used to it in time. They're good kids.

Therapist: How would you describe yourself as a person?

Patient: Interesting question. I would say I am joyful, appreciative, inquisitive, and helpful.

Therapist: Which of these four descriptors really captures the essence of who you are?

Patient: I would say the most important to me is the joyful.

Therapist: So what does "joyful" mean to you in terms of your sinuses condition? Right now you're experiencing a sinus headache. How does joyful characterize you at a time like this?

Patient: It means being pleasant and hopeful and trying to make the most of the situation. It means transcending the pain and being patient with myself and trying to learn something from this consultation.

Therapist: I appreciate how you handle yourself in a trying situation. Can you say a little bit more about what "joyful" means in your life?

Patient: It means waking up in the morning, feeling the warmth of the sun, hearing the birds sing, and visiting my new grandson. Life doesn't get any better than that! [*Smiles broadly*]

Therapist: If I were to ask your husband that same question of describing you as a person, what would he probably say?

This circular question is intended to further evaluate the nature and quality of her relationship with her husband, which likely reflects the quality of her objective relations.

Patient: I'm not sure I can answer precisely for him, but it would probably be something like this: helpful, loving, active, and hardworking. He knows I have my hands full and that I try to do too many things at one time. He's a really good man and he only wants the best for me.

Therapist: How would you describe your relationship with him?

Patient: It's very comfortable, caring, and loving.

Therapist: What's the impact of your symptoms on him?

Patient: He's a little worried. He'd like me to be better. He watches me engage in all these preventive measures and tries to give whatever help he can.

Therapist: If we can shift now to your earlier life, can you describe what it was like growing up in your family?

This led to an extended discussion about her bonding with her parents and queries about her family's values, dynamics, and religious and spiritual beliefs. It briefly assessed any history of abuse or neglect. She reports being an only child who felt deeply loved and cared for by both parents. Ellen recalls that her parents were kind and considerate and showed affection openly, and although they occasionally disagreed, they seemed to resolve issues quickly. She was expected to be considerate of others and find her passion in life and pursue it. For Ellen, that meant marrying her high school sweetheart, raising a family, and following her dream of becoming a hairstylist and maybe some day owning her own shop.

Therapist: So far, you have made some self-management efforts like diet modification, nasal irrigation, and so forth. They've helped a little, but apparently not as much as you had hoped. What other options are there?

Patient: Well, my doctor has ordered a CAT scan, and she said yes, my last course of antibiotics didn't make the difference; she would talk to me about surgery. She's hopeful.

Therapist: What if you are to hear that your condition was not going to get better but might even get progressively worse? What would that mean to you?

Patient: It would mean I would have to learn better coping skills.

Therapist: And in terms of your outlook of joyfulness?

Patient: I'd just keep going. In the big picture view of things, my life is good. I have people who love me and care about me and whom I care about, too. We also have a family that needs me to be there for them. I just keep looking and hoping to find ways of making my situation better. So I'd keep living with it with hopefulness.

Therapist: Researchers have found that there are two emotions that are commonly associated with chronic sinusitis. They are anger and resentment. Let's talk a bit about what part, if any, anger and resentment have in your life. What about anger?

Patient: Oh, I get angry every once in a while. Just this morning on the way here, a guy ran a red light and almost hit us. So I got a little angry.

Therapist: Say more about it. How intense and how long did it last?

Patient: Well, it was more of an annoyance and frustration. After all, there was no accident, nobody got hurt, and I recalled that had driven through a stop sign or two myself. So my frustration and anger only lasted about a minute or two.

Therapist: Is that a typical way in which you experience anger?

Patient:	Yes. I say so.
Therapist:	What about resentment?
Patient:	It's not really been a problem for me. I guess I'm pretty easy-going.

Although she appears to have a compulsive personality style with some dependent traits, there is no evidence of a personality disorder. Rather, she appears as a high-functioning individual whose family of origin and nuclear family appear to be very high functioning.

Therapist:	OK. Maybe we can now focus on some environmental factors and stressors and their impact on you. Now the city you live in, Chicago, is reportedly the third most polluted metropolitan area in the United States. So air pollution can be a major exacerbant for individuals with chronic sinusitis. Indoor air cleaners and negative-ion generators can be helpful to many with sinus problems.
Patient:	I think it could be very helpful for me. I've been reading about ion generators, and I will investigate further. The house we moved from 2 years ago had an air-cleaning system that covered the whole house. I could really tell the difference when we moved to our present house. I'm just wondering if the fact that my condition has gotten worse in the last year and a half has something to do with not having purified air in my present home. I think that it does. A few months ago, my husband and I talked about a full house air-cleaning system, but it's very expensive, and it may be possible in the future but not right now.
Therapist:	You mentioned that your sinus symptoms were worse at night and on awakening. Until you are in a position to install a master air purification unit in your house, what do you think of getting a room-size air purifier for your bedroom in the interim?
Patient:	Yes, I think it would be important, and I think we can afford it right now.
Therapist:	Also, what kind of chemicals are you exposed to in your work as a hairstylist?
Patient:	There are many. Hair dyes, hair sprays, and the chemicals for permanents. Those are probably the worst. It seems like I'm surrounded by those 8 hours a day. There are many propellants, which I know irritate my sinuses, in the products we use. And I've been trying to switch over to products without them.
Therapist:	How many hours a week a week are you at the shop?
Patient:	It's about 40 hours a week now . . . wait a minute; I used to work 20 hours a week, until about a year ago when I increased my

	hours. And that seems to coincide with the increase of my symptoms. Could that be important?
Therapist:	It sure could, because you've increased the dose of your exposure. Let me ask something else. Which days of the week do you work?
Patient:	Weekdays only: Monday to Friday.
Therapist:	Do you notice any difference in symptoms during the week as compared to weekends?
Patient:	Hmmm. I think they were worse in the middle of the week and better on the weekends. I've never thought about that before. Do you think that means that my exposure to chemicals at work is making the difference?
Therapist:	There is a good likelihood. Have you considered getting a portable air cleaner for your cubicle at your hair salon?
Patient:	No. But I think it would be a good experiment to try and see what difference it might make.

At this point, there is every indication that chemical and environmental exposures are key factors. There is no obvious indication for psychotherapy. However, health-focused counseling wherein recommendations are framed in terms of her psychological dynamics and are tailored to her current context does appear to be indicated. Accordingly, the session shifts to beginning this process and observing her response to it.

Therapist:	I agree. It would be a worthwhile experiment. [*Pause*] It does not appear that the emotional stressors play a major role in your chronic sinusitis, whereas environmental stressors, particularly air quality, seemed to have a prominent role. I also agree with you that physiological dynamics are critical in understanding your chronic sinusitis. The key is to control mucus production, since it is being overproduced largely in response to environmental exposure. So efforts to reduce exposure to chemicals and other air pollutants may go a long way in reducing mucus production. The other environmental stressor that can be addressed is diet. And I would encourage you to continue eliminating other foods that are mucous forming. And there are a number of specific nutrients that might help you. These are described in the chronic sinusitis self-management program called *Sinus Survival* [Ivker, 2000]. There is a book, pamphlets, and a Web site that have been useful to many persons like yourself. By the way, preliminary research shows this program to be quite effective even for individuals who have had no relief from multiple courses of antibiotics and/or surgeries.
Patient:	I've heard about the program, and I think I'm incorporating some parts of it right now. I have a friend who has been in-

volved in for about 3 months or so, and she says she is much better as a result. I'll check into it further.

Therapist: One possible reason you have not responded to antibiotics lately it is that the underlying pathogen or bug is not bacterial. It may well be a fungus or mold. And fungi do not respond to antibiotics. Fortunately, it is possible to identify and treat fungal infections.

Patient: That's very interesting. I didn't know that.

Therapist: So far, we've discussed a number of internal and external stressors that can trigger or exacerbate your sinusitis. First are the internal stressors, including negative attitudes and a sense of drivenness and compulsivity, and a caring social support system. You seem to have positive attitudes, particularly a joyful attitude, and a caring support system, including your husband, children, and grandchildren, which I believe serve as important health resources or coping resources against disease and illness. Second are the external or environmental stressors. It seems that air quality both in your home and at your job are exacerbants. You are to be commended for your efforts to modify your diet. But you probably shouldn't be disheartened because those diet modifications didn't clear up your condition entirely. Most individuals with years of chronic sinusitis symptoms did not achieve total remission or near total remission of their symptoms just by making changes in one aspect of their life, such as diet, or with one or two new health behaviors, such as nasal irrigation or steaming. By definition, a chronic illness involves multiple causes and exacerbants and so requires multiple interventions. Thus, there are several environmental stressors that cause or exacerbate symptoms; each of those stressors needs to be addressed. In your case, this means reducing or eliminating exposure to chemicals and propellants at your workplace, and whatever triggers or exacerbants there are in your sleeping quarters.

Patient: I agree that I have been expecting that one or two changes would make all the difference. And they haven't. I'm thinking now that I really haven't addressed the exposure issue at home and at work. And I really need to.

Therapist: Say a little more about that, if you will—about your coworkers. Do any of them have similar symptoms or concerns?

Patient: [Pause] As a matter of fact, I think some have. I notice that three or four women are taking over-the-counter sinus medicines regularly. We've talked on and off about our symptoms. I don't think anyone is as bad as I am, yet. But now that I think about it, none of the others had sinus problems before they began working as hairstylists. You know, it may be that chemical exposure is the common link.

Therapist: It may well be. Here's a hypothetical for you: What if, after you were able to reduce your exposure at work to chemicals and propellants, your symptoms didn't improve appreciably? What options would you have at that point?

Patient: That's a tall question. I guess one option is to find another line of work. But I hope it doesn't have to be that way, because I really like what I do, and I am good at it. It is really going to be important for me to find other, safer hair products and install an air purifier. Who knows, maybe we could think about installing a central air purification system in the whole salon. Besides being good for the staff, it would also be good for our customers.

Therapist: What criteria have you used in the past to make decisions about dealing with your sinusitis?

Patient: Well, probably they have been cost and ease of use.

Therapist: Those two criteria seem to be logical criteria. Decisions are also made based on emotional criteria. What might yours be, and how much weight would you give to them?

Patient: My main criterion would be respect for my body. And my sense is that if a job is harmful to me, then I would choose health rather than stay in that job. The thing about cost would be secondary. And I think my husband would agree.

Therapist: OK. [*Pause*] Before we go on, do you have a question or comment?

Patient: No question but a comment. It's a lot clearer to me now that there are many causes and triggers to my sinusitis, and so it's not realistic to think that just one or two changes in my life will make all the difference. I've never really put much thought into how air quality and my exposure to chemicals at work and how dust mites and whatever else is in our bedroom, how they affect me. It's become clearer that I need to address these things. I now see that I have another option or options other than surgery. So this has been very helpful. I think I know what needs to be done. Is this something you can help me with further?

The session concludes with a discussion of a disposition plan.

REVIEW OF THE COMPREHENSIVE ASSESSMENT

The comprehensive assessment was completed in a 90-minute face-to-face session. In addition, I reviewed the clinical case report from her ear, nose, and throat (ENT) specialist, which indicated that Ellen's extensive history of treatment use worsened in the past several years and noted the various antibiotic trials as well as the self-management programs in which she had been involved and that sinus surgery seemed to be the only remaining option. The report indicated that Ellen was a delightful and cooperative patient who was very conscientious about the specialist's treatment regimen and her self-management program. The patient's desire for a second opinion was well warranted, because research indicates that such surgery has only a limited to moderate likelihood of achieving resolution of symptoms in the long term (Ivker, 2000). Besides medical treatment, she had not received any prior counseling or psychotherapeutic services. It is interesting to note that the patient was open to psychotherapeutic intervention if that was indicated.

The goal of this consultation was to comprehensively assess relevant biopsychosocial dynamics and functioning related to her chronic illness. It was noted that her level of illness progression was moderately severe, although the impact of her respiratory condition only mildly impacted her personal and work life. She rarely was unable to attend to household responsibilities, and even on days in which she was experiencing a splitting sinus headache, she would go to her job because she didn't want to disappoint her clients who had long-standing appointments with her. Although her explanatory model of her illness is scientifically accurate and did account, in part, for environmental exposure, it did not include chemical exposure. Her health behaviors were consistent with the self-management program established by the ENT clinic, and her compliance with the program was considered to be excellent. A significant finding of the assessment was the extent of exposure to hydrocarbons and other caustic chemicals at her job, which seem the likely explanation for her increased symptoms in the past year; 11 months ago, Ellen increased her hours from 20 to 40 per week at her hair salon job, which meant doubling her exposure to chemicals, which appeared to intensify her symptoms. Her early parental bond appears to have been quite secure—that is, loving and caring—with no indication of abuse or neglect. Her schemas about self and the world were positive and health promoting, as was her family narrative. Her personality style is characterized as obsessive–compulsive and dependent, and she is one of the rare individuals who grew up in a family functioning at the optimal level, with a Global Assessment of Relationship Functioning (GARF; American Psychiatric Association, 2000) score of 90+ (Beavers & Hampson, 1990). Her religious and spiritual beliefs were positive and health sustaining. Her resources were judged to be very adequate, and she appeared to possess well-developed self-capacities. Her readiness for treatment was clearly high, that is, at the action stage. Similarly, her capacity for self-management was very high, as reported by the ENT clinic. As noted by her physician, Ellen has demonstrated a consistently high level of adequacy for engaging in a treatment relationship with health care providers. As evidenced by her responsivity to the initial interventions, particularly in the

TABLE 9.1
Summary of Key Assessment Factors for the Case of Ellen

Assessment factor	Maximum responsiveness
Level of illness progression and impact	Moderate and mild
Illness representation or explanatory model	Realistic
Adequacy of health behaviors and exposure Hx	Positive; chemicals at job
Early parental bond and ACE (abuse or neglect)	Healthy, secure bond; none
Personal schemas and family narratives	Health prone
Personality style or disorder	Style: obsessive–compulsive and dependent
Family competence and style	Highly functional; integrated
Religious and spiritual beliefs	Positive
Patient resources, especially self-capacities	Very adequate; developed
Readiness for treatment or capacity for self-mgmt	High—action stage; high
Adequacy of Tx relationship with other providers	High
Alignment of explanatory model and treatment goals	High
Phase of illness	Phase 3, possibly Phase 4

Note. Hx = history; ACE = adverse childhood experience; self-mgmt = self-management; Tx = treatment.

discussion of the impact of the workplace chemical exposure explanatory model, the alignment of the patient–therapist explanatory model and treatment goals should be high. Finally, it appeared that Ellen is in Phase 3 of her illness. Because there are some indications that she has already integrated some aspects of her daily life into a new self, she is moving into Phase 4. In short, there is every indication that she is functioning at a high level of wellness, even while her health status is compromised. Table 9.1 summarizes key factors of the comprehensive assessment.

CASE CONCEPTUALIZATION

On the basis of the comprehensive assessment, it appears that this case can be conceptualized rather succinctly: Ellen's increased exposure to noxious chemicals used at her hair salon appear to account for her significant increase in symptoms and further progression of her chronic illness. Despite all the lifestyle and diet modifications she had initiated—that is, her adherence to the sinus self-management program and her compliance with several trials of antibiotic therapy and alternative medicine interventions—it appears that she could not mount a sufficient immune response to that increased chemical exposure. Although she is a positive person, is quite mature psychologically, appears to have a highly supportive family and social system, and is effectively beginning to integrate her chronic illness as one part of her self-conception, chemical exposure is a key element in negatively impacting her health status.

TREATMENT ISSUES

On the basis of the case conceptualization, reducing exposure to workplace chemicals and other environmental exposures should be a major treatment target. Accordingly, a follow-up plan was established that included the following short-term goals, which were mutually set: (a) reduce workplace chemical exposure by replacing styling gels and permanent solutions with less toxic products; (b) add an air purifier; and (c) incorporate the Sinus Survival protocol (Ivker, 2000) to her self-management program. A follow-up appointment was scheduled in 1 month, and we agreed to meet again in 3 to 4 months, depending on the need to do so.

CONCLUDING NOTE

When it is clear that psychotherapists are evaluating patients, such as Ellen, with chronic illness who have relatively circumscribed illness parameters that are not compounded by significant psychological and social dynamics, a pattern analysis is usually not necessary. The value of the comprehensive assessment is that it is an in-depth exploration of a patient's entire life space. Although it may seem surprising that no one in the ENT clinic identified Ellen's increasing exposure to workplace chemicals, the reality is that, unless patients volunteer information or are asked about changes in their daily routines, increased hours of chemical exposure is not considered in the relatively limited assessment protocols used by many medical personnel. In this case, it happened to be a biological factor, but it just as easily could have been a social factor, that is, increased stressors associated with financial problems, the potential for job loss, or a child with a life-threatening illness. Or, as recent research has pointed out, there is widespread underrecognition of the impact of early childhood abuse as an etiological factor or exacerbant of a chronic disease, as well as a lack of recognition of its impact on adherence to treatment. Unless clinicians ask and elicit such a history, case conceptualizations and treatment plans cannot be appropriately informed and complete. For that reason, comprehensive assessments are essential in working with any patient presenting with a chronic illness, and clinicians who incorporate a biopsychosocial perspective provide a much-needed and much-appreciated service. Finally, working with and being able to assist patients like Ellen in making small strategic changes that can have significant long-range positive consequences for their health and well-being can be very satisfying and inspiring for psychotherapists and other clinicians.

REFERENCES

Adler, A. (1956). *The individual psychology of Alfred Adler: A systematic presentation in selections from his writings* (H. L. Ansbacher & R. R. Ansbacher, Eds.). New York: Harper & Row.

Ansbacher, H., & Ansbacher, R. (Eds.). (1956). *The individual psychology of Alfred Adler.* New York: Harper & Row.

American Psychiatric Association. (1994). *Diagnostic and statistical manual of mental disorders* (4th ed.). Washington, DC: Author.

American Psychiatric Association. (2000). *Diagnostic and statistical manual of mental disorders* (4th ed., text rev.). Washington, DC: Author.

Angel, R. J., & Williams, K. (2001). Cultural models of health and illness. In I. Cuellar & F. A. Paniagua (Eds.), *Handbook of multicultural mental health* (pp. 25–44). San Diego, CA: Academic Press.

Arredondo, P. (1996). MCT theory and Latina(o)-American populations. In D. W. Sue, A. E. Ivey, & P. B. Pedersen (Eds.), *A theory of multicultural counseling and therapy* (pp. 217–235). Pacific Grove, CA: Brooks/Cole.

Bandura, A. (1997). *Self-efficacy.* New York: Freeman.

Baum, A., & Andersen, B. L. (Eds.). (2001). *Psychosocial interventions for cancer.* Washington, DC: American Psychological Association.

Beavers, W. R., & Hampson, R. (1990). *Successful families: Assessment and intervention.* New York: Norton.

Beers, M. (2003). *The Merck manual of medical information* (2nd ed.). New York: Pocket Books.

Beers, M., & Berkow, R. (Eds.). (1999). *The Merck manual of diagnosis and therapy* (17th ed.). New York: Wiley.

Beitman, B. (1987). *The structure of individual psychotherapy.* New York: Guilford Press.

Beitman, B. (1993). Pharmacotherapy and the stages of psychotherapeutic change. In J. M. Oldham, M. B. Riba, & A. Tasman (Eds.), *American Psychiatric Press review of psychiatry,* (Vol. 12, pp. 521–540). Washington, DC: American Psychiatric Press.

Binder, J. (2004). *Key competencies in brief dynamics psychotherapy: Clinical practice beyond the manual.* New York: Guilford Press.

Bishop, G. (1998). East meets West: Illness cognition and behavior in Singapore. *Applied Psychology: An International Review, 47,* 519–534.

Blanchard, E. B. (2001). *Irritable bowel syndrome: Psychosocial assessment and treatment.* Washington, DC: American Psychological Association.

Blanchard, E. B., & Malamood, M. (1996). Psychological treatment of irritable bowel syndrome. *Professional Psychology: Research and Practice, 27,* 241–245.

Blanchard, E. B., & Scharff, J. (2002). Psychosocial aspects of assessment and treatment of irritable bowel syndrome in adults and recurrent abdominal pain in children. *Journal of Consulting and Clinical Psychology, 70,* 725–739.

Brown, L., Kessel, S., Lourie, K., Ford, H., & Lipsitt, L. (1997). Influence of sexual abuse on HIV-related attitudes and behaviors in adolescent psychiatric inpatients. *Journal of the American Academy of Child and Adolescent Psychiatry, 36,* 316–322.

Buchi, S., Villiger, P., Kauer, Y., Klaghofer, R., Sensky, T., & Stoll, T. (2000). PRISM (Pictorial Representation of Illness and Self Measure)—A novel visual method to assess the global burden of illness in patients with systemic lupus erythematosus. *Lupus, 9,* 368–373.

Canino, G., & Guarnaccia, P. (1997). Methodological challenges in the assessment of Hispanic children and adolescents. *Applied Developmental Science, 1,* 124–134.

Centers for Disease Control and Prevention. (2002). *The burden of diseases and their risk factors.* National Center for Chronic Disease Prevention and Health Promotion. Atlanta, GA: Author.

Chamie, M. (1995). What does morbidity have to do with disability? *Disability and Rehabilitation, 17,* 323–337.

Chesler, M. A., & Yoak, M. (1984). Self-help groups for parents of children with cancer. In H. B. Roback (Ed.), *Helping patients and their families cope with medical problems: A guide to therapeutic group work in clinical settings* (pp. 481–526). San Francisco: Jossey-Bass.

Cioffi, D. (1991). Beyond attentional strategies: A cognitive–perceptual model of somatic interpretation. *Psychological Bulletin, 109,* 25–41.

Clark, A. (2002). *Early recollections: Theory and practice in counseling and psychotherapy.* New York: Brunner-Routledge.

Crawford, I., & Fishman, B. (1997). *Psychosocial interventions in HIV disease: A stage-focused and culture specific approach (cognitive–behavioral therapy).* New York: Jason Aronson.

Didjurgeit, U., Kruse, J., Schmitz, N., Stuckenschneider, P., & Sawicki, T. (2002). A time-limited, problem-orientated psychotherapeutic intervention in Type 1 diabetic patients with complications: A randomized controlled trial. *Diabetic Medicine, 19,* 814–822.

Digeronimo, T. (2002). *New hope for people with lupus.* New York: Prima.

Dreikurs, R. (1967). *Psychodynamics: Psychotherapy and counseling.* Chicago: Alfred Adler Institute.

Dunkel-Schetter, C., & Wortman, C. B. (1982). The interpersonal dynamics of cancer: Problems in social relationships and their impact on the patient. In H. S. Friedman, & M. R. DiMatteo (Eds.), *Interpersonal issues in health care* (pp. 69–100). New York: Academic Press.

Dunn, H. (1961). *High-level wellness.* Arlington, VA: R. W. Beatty.

Edwards, V., Anda, R., Felitti, V., & Dube, S. (2004). Adverse childhood experiences and health-related quality of life as an adult. In K. Kendall-Tackett (Ed.),

Health consequences of abuse in the family: A clinical guide for evidence-based practice (pp. 81–94). Washington, DC: American Psychological Association.

Edwards, V., Anda, R., Gu, D., & Felitti, V. (2000, November). *The relation between childhood use and smoking persistence in adults with smoking-related symptoms and diseases.* Paper presented at the 14th National Chronic Disease Conference, Dallas, TX.

Eells, T., & Lombart, K. (2003). Case formulation and treatment concepts among novice, experienced, and expert cognitive–behavioral and psychodynamics therapists. *Psychotherapy Research, 13,* 187–204.

Eimer, B., & Freeman, A. (1999). *Pain management psychotherapy: A practical guide.* New York: Wiley.

Eisenberg, M. G. (1984). Spinal cord injuries. In H. B. Roback (Ed.), *Helping patients and their families cope with medical problems: A guide to therapeutic group work in clinical settings* (pp. 107–129). San Francisco: Jossey-Bass.

Engel, G. (1977, April 8). The need for a new medical model: A challenge to biomedical science. *Science, 196,* 129–136.

Erlen, J. (2002). Ethics in chronic illness. In P. D. Larsen & I. M. Lubkin (Eds.), *Chronic illness: Impact and interventions,* (5th ed., pp. 407–429). Sudbury, MA: Jones and Bartlett.

Euster, S. (1984). Adjusting to an adult family member's cancer. In H. B. Roback (Ed.), *Helping patients and their families cope with medical problems: A guide to therapeutic group work in clinical settings* (pp. 428–452). San Francisco: Jossey-Bass.

Felitti, V., Anda, R., Nordenberg, D., Williamson, D., Spitz, A., Edwards, V., et al. (1998). Relationship of childhood abuse and household dysfunction to many of the leading causes of death in adults. *American Journal of Preventive Medicine, 14,* 245–258.

Fennell, P. (2001). *The chronic illness workbook.* Oakland, CA: New Harbinger.

Fennell, P. (2003). *Managing chronic illness using the four-phase treatment approach.* Hoboken, NJ: Wiley.

Finkelhor, D. (1994). Current information on the scope and nature of child sexual abuse. *Future of Children, 4,* 31–53.

Folkman, S., & Greer, S. (2000). Promoting psychological well-being in the face of serious illness: When theory, research, and practice inform each other. *Psycho-Oncology, 9,* 11–19.

Friedberg, F., & Jason, L. A. (1998). *Understanding chronic fatigue: An empirical guide to assessment and treatment.* Washington, DC: American Psychological Association.

Friedman, H. S., & DiMatteo, M. R. (1989). *Health psychology.* Englewood Cliffs, NJ: Prentice Hall.

Fukuda, K., Straus, S. E., Hickie, I., Sharpre, M. C., Dobbins, J. G., & Komaroff, A. (1994). The chronic fatigue syndrome: A comprehensive approach to its definition and study. *Annals of Internal Medicine, 121,* 953–959.

Gardner-Nix, J., Dupak, K., & Lam-McCulloch, J. (2004). Comparison of PRISM (Pictorial Representation of Illness and Self-Measure) scores and the SF–36 quality of life questionnaire to assess suffering in chronic non-cancer pain patients. *Journal of Pain, 5*(3, Suppl. 1).

Garrett, M., & Myers, J. (1996). The rule of opposites: A paradigm for counseling Native Americans. *Journal of Multicultural Counseling and Development, 24*, 89–104.

Gelso, C., & Hayes, J. (2002). The management of countertransferences. In J. Norcross (Ed.), *Psychotherapy relationships that work: Therapist contributions and responsiveness to patients* (pp. 267–284). New York: Oxford University Press.

Gonder-Frederick, L., Cox, D., & Ritterband, L. (2002). Diabetes and behavioral medicine: The second decade. *Journal of Consulting and Clinical Psychology, 70*, 611–625.

Goodheart, C. D., & Lansing, M. H. (1996). *Treating people with chronic disease: A psychological guide.* Washington, DC: American Psychological Association.

Hagglund, K., Halley, W., Reveille, J., & Alacren, G. (1989). Predicting individual differences in pain and functional impairment among patients with rheumatoid arthritics. *Arthritis and Rheumatism, 32*, 851–858.

Hamburg, D. A., Elliott, G. R., & Parron, D. L. (1982). *Health and behavior: Frontiers of research in the biobehavioral sciences.* Washington, DC: National Academy Press.

Harper, R. (2003). *Personality-guided therapy in behavioral medicine.* Washington, DC: American Psychological Association.

Haven, T., & Pearlman, L. (2004). Minding the body: The intersection of dissociation and physical health in relational trauma psychotherapy. In K. Kendall-Tackett (Ed.), *Health consequences of abuse in the family: A clinical guide for evidence-based practice* (pp. 215–232). Washington, DC: American Psychological Association.

Heijmans, M., Foets, M., Rijken, M., Schreurs, K., de Ridder, D., & Bensing, J. (2001). Stress in chronic disease: Do the perceptions of patients and their general practitioners match? *British Journal of Health Psychology, 6*, 229–243.

Hendrick, S. S. (1985). Behavioral medicine approaches to diabetes mellitus. In N. Schneiderman & J. T. Tapp (Eds.), *Behavioral medicine: The biopsychosocial approach* (pp. 509–531). Hillsdale, NJ: Erlbaum.

Hettler, W. (1984). Wellness: Encouraging a lifetime pursuit of excellence. *Health Values, 8*, 13–17.

Institute of Medicine, Committee on Rapid Advance Demonstration Projects: Health Care Finance and Delivery Systems. (2002, November 19). In J. M. Corrigan, A. Greiner, & S. M. Erickson (Eds.), *Fostering rapid advances in health care: Learning from system demonstrations.* Washington, DC: The National Academies Press.

Ivker, R. (2000). *Sinus survival: The holistic medical treatment for allergies, cold, and sinusitis* (4th ed.). New York: Tarcher/Putnam.

Johnson, S. B. (1985). The family and the child with chronic illness. In D. C. Turk & R. D. Kerns (Eds.), *Health, illness, and families: A life-span perspective* (pp. 220–254). New York: Wiley.

Johnson, S. B. (2002). *Emotionally focused couple therapy with trauma survivors: Strengthening attachment bonds.* New York: Guilford Press.

Jordan-Marsh, M., Gilbert, J., Ford, J., & Kleeman, C. (1984). Life-style intervention: A conceptual framework. *Patient Education and Counseling, 6,* 29–38.

Joung, I., van de Mheen, H., Stronks, K., van Poppel, F., & Machenbach, J. (1998). A longitudinal study of health selection in marital transitions. *Social Science and Medicine, 46,* 425–435.

Kapust, L. R., & Weintraub, S. (1984). Living with a family member suffering from Alzheimer's disease. In H. B. Roback (Ed.), *Helping patients and their families cope with medical problems* (pp. 453–480). San Francisco: Jossey-Bass.

Kellner, R. (1986). *Somatization and hypochondriasis.* New York: Praeger Publishers.

Kendall-Tackett, K. (2003). *Treating the long-term health effects of childhood abuse: A guide for mental health, medical, and social service professionals.* New York: Civic Research Institute.

Kendall-Tackett, K., & Marshall, R. (1999). Victimization and diabetes: An exploratory study. *Child Abuse and Neglect, 23,* 593–596.

Kerns, R. D., & Curley, A. D. (1985). A biopsychosocial approach to illness and the family: Neurological diseases across the life span. In D. C. Turk & R. D. Kerns (Eds.), *Health, illness, and families: A life-span perspective* (pp. 146–182). New York: Wiley.

Kleinman, A. (1988). *Rethinking psychiatry: From cultural category to personal experience.* New York: Free Press.

Kleinman, A., Eisenberg, L., & Good, B. (1978). Culture, illness, and care. *Annals of Internal Medicine, 88,* 251–258.

Lambert, M., & Ogles, B. (2003). The efficacy and effectiveness of psychotherapy. In M. Lambert (Ed.), *Bergin and Garfield's handbook of psychotherapy and behavior change* (5th ed.). New York: Wiley.

Lane, N. (2003). A unifying view of ageing and disease: The double-agent theory. *Journal of Theoretical Biology, 225,* 531–540.

Lazarus, R., & Folkman, S. (1984). *Stress, appraisal, and coping.* New York: Springer Publishing Company.

Leong, F. T. L., Wager, N. S., & Tata, S. P. (1995). Racial and ethnic variations in help-seeking attitudes. In J. G. Ponterotto, J. M. Casas, L. M. Suzuki, & C. M. Alexander (Eds.), *Handbook of multicultural counseling* (pp. 415–438). Thousand Oaks, CA: Sage.

Levant, R. (2004). 21st century psychology: Toward a biopsychosocial model. *Psychotherapy Bulletin, 39,* 2, 8–11.

Leventhal, H., Diefenbach, M., & Levanthal, E. (1992). Illness cognition: Using common sense to understand treatment adherence and affect in cognitive interactions. *Cognitive Therapy and Research, 16,* 143–163.

Leventhal, H., Levanthal, E., & Cameron, L. (2000). Representation, procedures, and affect in illness self-regulation: A perceptual–cognitive model. In A. Baum,

T. Revenson, & J. Singer (Eds.), *Handbook of health psychology* (pp. 19–47). Mahwah, NJ: Erlbaum.

Lewis, M. (2002). *Multicultural health counseling: Special topics acknowledging diversity.* Boston: Allyn & Bacon.

Linehan, M. (1993). *Cognitive–behavioral treatment of borderline personality disorder.* New York: Guilford Press.

Lubkin, I., & Larsen, P. (2002). What is chronicity? In I. Lubkin & P. Larsen (Eds.), *Chronic illness: Impact and interventions.* (5th ed., pp. 3–24). Sudbury, MA: Jones and Bartlett.

Lustman, P., & Clouse, R. (2002). Treatment of depression in diabetes: Impact on mood and medical outcome. *Journal of Psychosomatic Research, 53,* 917–925.

Mamby, S. (2004). The spectrum of victimization and the implications for health. In K. Kendall-Tackett (Ed.), *Health consequences of abuse in the family: A clinical guide for evidence-based practice* (pp. 7–27). Washington, DC: American Psychological Association.

Marsella, A. J., & Yamada, A. M. (2001). Culture and mental health: An introduction and overview of foundations, concepts, and issues. In I. Cuellar & F. A. Paniagua (Eds.), *Handbook of multicultural mental health* (pp. 3–24). San Diego, CA: Academic Press.

McCauley, J., Kern, D., Kolodner, K., Dill, L., Schroeder, A., DeChant, H., et al. (1997). Clinical characteristics of women with a history of childhood abuse: Unhealed wounds. *Journal of the American Medical Association, 277,* 1362–1368.

McGinnis, J., Williams-Russo, P., & Knickman, J. (2002). The case for more active policy attention to health promotion. *Health Affairs, 21,* 78–93.

McMillan, H., Fleming, J., Trocme, N., Boyle, M., Wong, M., Racine, Y., et al. (1997). Prevalence of child physical and sexual abuse in the community: Results from the Ontario Health Supplement. *Journal of the American Medical Association, 278,* 131–135.

Melzack, R. (1980). Psychological aspects of pain. In J. Bonica (Ed.), *Pain* (pp. 277–299). New York: Raven Press.

Meyer, A., & Lewis, D. (1994). *The child with chronic illness* (American Family Physician Monograph No. 182). Kansas City, MO: American Academy of Family Physicians.

Miller, W. R., & Rollnick, S. (2002). *Motivational interviewing: Preparing people for change* (2nd ed.). New York: Guilford Press.

Millon, T. (1981). *Personality and its disorders: DSM–III, Axis II.* New York: Wiley.

Millon, T. (1999). *Personality guided therapy.* New York: Wiley.

Millon, T., Antoni, M., Millon, C., Mengher, R., & Grossman, S. (2001). *Millon Behavioral Health Inventory Diagnostic Manual.* Eagen, MN: Pearson Assessments.

Millon, T., & Everly, G. (1985). *Disorders of personality.* New York: Wiley.

Millon, T., Green, C., & Meagher, R. (1982). *Millon Behavioral Health Inventory manual.* Minneapolis, MN: National Computer Systems.

Monat, A., & Lazarus, R. (1991). Introduction: Stress and coping: Some current issues and controversies. In A. Monat & R. Lazarus (Eds.), *Stress and coping: An anthology* (3rd ed., pp. 1–15). New York: Columbia University Press.

Moorey, S., & Greer, S. (2003). *Cognitive behaviour therapy for people with cancer* (2nd ed.). New York: Oxford University Press.

Moran, G., Fonagy, P., Kurtz, A., Bolton, A., & Brook, C. (1991). A controlled study of the psychoanalytic treatment of brittle diabetes. *Journal of the American Academy of Child & Adolescent Psychiatry, 30,* 926–935.

Moss-Morris, R., Weinman, J., Petrie, K., Horne, R., Cameron, L., & Buick, D. (2002). The Revised Illness Perception Questionnaire (IPQ–R). *Psychology and Health, 7,* 1–16.

Mukherji, B. (1995). Cross-cultural issues in illness and wellness: Implications for depression. *Journal of Social Distress and the Homeless, 4,* 203–217.

Myers, J., Sweeney, T., & Witmer, J. (2000). The wheel of wellness: Counseling for wellness. *Journal of Counseling and Development, 78,* 251–266.

National Center for Chronic Disease Prevention and Health Promotion. (2000). *Chronic diseases and their risk factors: The nation's leading causes of death, 1999.* Washington, DC: Author.

Nicassio, P. M., & Smith, T. W. (1995). *Managing chronic illness: A biopsychosocial perspective.* Washington, DC: American Psychological Association.

Norcross, J. (2002). Empirically supported therapy relationships. In J. Norcross (Ed.). *Psychotherapy relationships that work: Therapist contributions and responsiveness to patients* (pp. 3–16). New York: Oxford University Press.

Pavlou, M. (1984). Multiple sclerosis. In H. B. Roback (Ed.), *Helping patients and their families cope with medical problems: A guide to therapeutic group work in clinical settings* (pp. 331–365). San Francisco: Jossey-Bass.

Pearlman, L. (1998). Trauma and the self: A theoretical and clinical perspective. *Journal of Emotional Abuse, 1,* 7–25.

Perera, F. (1997, November 7). Environment and cancer: Who are susceptible? *Science, 278,* 1068–1073.

Pilch, J. (1985). *Wellness spirituality.* New York: Crossroad.

Ponika, J., Sherris, D., & Kern, E. (1999). The diagnosis and incidence of allergic fungal sinusitis. *Mayo Clinic Proceedings, 74,* 877–884.

Prochaska, J., Norcross, J., & DiClemente, C. (1994). *Changing for good.* New York: Morrow.

Raine, R., Haines, A., Sensky, T., Hutchings, A., Larkin, K., & Black, N. (2002). Systematic review of mental health interventions for patients with common somatic symptoms: Can research evidence from secondary care be extrapolated to primary care? *British Medical Journal, 325,* 1082–1086.

Redman, B. (2004). *Patient self-management of chronic disease: The health care provider's challenge.* Sudbury, MA: Jones and Bartlett.

Robert Wood Johnson Foundation. (1994). *Annual report: Health in the United States, 1994.* New York: Author.

Russek, L., & Schwartz, G. (1996). Narrative descriptions of parental love and caring predict health status in midlife: A 35-year follow-up of the Harvard Mastery of Stress Study. *Alternative Therapies in Health and Medicine, 2,* 55–62.

Russek, L., & Schwartz, G. (1997a). Perceptions of parental caring predict health status in midlife: A 35-year follow-up of the Harvard Mastery of Stress Study. *Psychosomatic Medicine, 59*, 144–149.

Russek, L., & Schwartz, G. (1997b). Feelings of parental caring predict health status in midlife: A 35-year follow-up of the Harvard Mastery of Stress Study. *Journal of Behavioral Medicine, 20*, 1–13.

Sadovsky, R. (2002). Cognitive behavior treatment of chronic disease. *American Family Physician, 65*, 1934.

Schiaffino, K., Shawaryn, J., & Blum, D. (1998). Examining the impact of illness representations on psychological adjustment to chronic illnesses. *Health Psychology, 17*, 262–268.

Schilling, L., Grey, M., & Knafl, K. (2002). The concept of self-management of Type 1 diabetes in children and adolescents: An evolutionary concept analysis. *Journal of Advanced Nursing, 37*, 87–99.

Schmidt, S., Wuetrich-Martone, O., & Nachtigall, C. (2002). Attachment and coping with chronic disease. *Journal of Psychosomatic Research, 7*, 1–22.

Segal, Z., Toner, B., Emmott, S., & Myran, D. (2000). *Cognitive–behavioral treatment of irritable bowel syndrome: The brain–gut connection.* New York: Guilford Press.

Sharoff, K. (2004). *Coping skills manual for treating chronic and terminal illness.* New York: Springer Publishing Company.

Siegel, D. (1999). *The developing mind: How relationships and the brain interact to shape who we are.* New York: Guilford Press.

Smyth, J., & Stone, A. (1999). Effects of writing about stressful experiences in symptom reduction in patients with asthma or rheumatoid arthritis: A randomized trial. *Journal of the American Medical Association, 281*, 1304–1309.

Snoek, D., van der Ven, C., & Lubach, C. (1999). Cognitive–behavioral group training for poorly controlled Type 1 diabetes patients: A psychoeducational approach. *Diabetes Spectrum, 12*, 147.

Sperry L. (1988). Biopsychosocial therapy: An integrative approach for tailoring treatment. *Individual Psychology, 44*, 225–235.

Sperry, L. (1995a). *Handbook of the diagnosis and treatment of DSM–IV personality disorders.* New York: Brunner/Mazel.

Sperry, L. (1995b). *Psychopharmacology and psychotherapy: Maximizing treatment outcomes.* New York: Brunner/Mazel.

Sperry, L. (1999a). Biopsychosocial therapy. *Journal of Individual Psychology, 55*, 233–247.

Sperry, L. (1999b). *Cognitive behavior therapy of the DSM–IV personality disorders: Highly effective interventions for the most common personality disorders.* Philadelphia: Brunner/Mazel.

Sperry, L. (2000). Biopsychosocial therapy: Essential strategies and tactics. In J. Carlson & L. Sperry (Eds.), *Brief therapy with individuals and couples.* Phoenix, AZ: Zeig, Tucker & Theisen.

Sperry, L. (2001a). The biological dimension in biopsychosocial therapy: Theory and clinical applications with couples. *Journal of Individual Psychology, 57*, 310–317.

Sperry, L. (2001b). Biopsychosocial therapy with individuals and couples: Integrative theory and interventions. In L. Sperry (Ed.), *Integrative and biopsychosocial therapy: Maximizing treatment outcomes with individuals and couples* (pp. 67–99). Alexandria, VA: American Counseling Association.

Sperry, L. (2003a). *Handbook of the diagnosis and treatment of the DSM–IV personality disorders* (2nd ed.). New York: Brunner-Routledge.

Sperry, L. (2003b). Integrative spiritually oriented psychotherapy: A case study of spiritual and psychological transformation. In P. Richards & A. Bergin (Eds.), *Casebook for a spiritual strategy in counseling and psychotherapy* (pp. 141–152). Washington, DC: American Psychological Association.

Sperry, L. (2005). Case conceptualizations: The missing link between theory and practice. *The Family Journal: Counseling and Therapy for Couples and Families, 13*, 71–76.

Sperry, L., Blackwell, B., Gudeman, J., & Faulkner, K. (1992). *Psychiatric case formulations.* Washington, DC: American Psychiatric Press.

Sperry, L., Brill, P., Howard, K., & Grissom, G. (1996). *Treatment outcomes in psychotherapy and psychiatric interventions.* New York: Brunner/Mazel.

Sperry, L., Carlson, J., & Kjos, D. (2003). *Becoming an effective therapist.* Boston: Allyn & Bacon.

Sperry, L., Lewis, J., Carlson, J., & Englar-Carlson, M. (2005). *Health promotion and health counseling: Effective counseling and psychotherapeutic strategies.* Boston: Allyn & Bacon.

Stein, M., & Barrett-Connor, E. (2000). Sexual assault and physical health: Findings from a population-based study of older adults. *Psychosomatic Medicine, 62*, 838–843.

Stone, M. (1993). *Abnormalities of personality: Within and beyond the realm of treatment.* New York: Norton.

Thomas, A., & Chess, S. (1977). *Temperament and development.* New York: Brunner/Mazel.

Thorn, B. (2004). *Cognitive therapy for chronic pain: A step-by-step guide.* New York: Guilford Press.

Turk, D. C., & Kerns, R. D. (1985). The family in health and illness. In D. C. Turk & R. D. Kerns (Eds.), *Health, illness, and families: A life-span perspective* (pp. 1–22). New York: Wiley.

Van der Poel, C. (1999). *Wholeness and holiness: A Christian response to human suffering.* Franklin, WI: Sheed & Ward.

Vingerhoets, A. (2004a). The Pictorial Representation of Self Measure and Illness Revised (PRISM–R): Measuring treatment outcome in whiplash patients. *Journal of Psychosomatic Research, 56*, 669.

Vingerhoets, A. (2004b). The PRISM–R: A pilot study among different patient groups. *Journal of Psychosomatic Research, 56,* 625.

Walker, J., Jackson, H., & Littlejohn, G. (2004). Models of adjustment to chronic illness: Using the example of rheumatoid arthritis. *Clinical Psychology Review, 24,* 461–488.

Wall, P., & Melzack, R. (1989). *The challenge of pain* (2nd ed). Hammondworth, England: Penguin.

Wallston, K. A., Wallston, B. S., & Devellis, R. (1978). Development of the Multidimensional Health Locus of Control (MHLOC) scales. *Health Education Monographs, 6,* 160–170.

Wallston, K. A., Stein, M., & Smith, C. (1994). Form C of the MHLC scales: A condition-specific measure of locus of control. *Journal of Personality Assessment, 63,* 534–553.

Wampold, B. (2001). *The great psychotherapy debate: Models, methods, and findings.* Mahwah, NJ: Erlbaum.

Weinman, J., Petrie, K., Moss-Morris, R., & Horne, R. (1996). The Illness Perception Questionnaire: A new method for assessing the cognitive representation of illness. *Psychology and Health, 11,* 431–455.

White, C. A. (2001). *Cognitive behaviour therapy for chronic medical problems: A guide to assessment and treatment in practice.* New York: Wiley.

White, M., & Epston, D. (1990). *Narrative means to therapeutic ends.* New York: Norton.

Winterowd, C., Beck, A., & Gruener, D. (2004). *Cognitive therapy with chronic pain patients.* New York: Springer Publishing Company.

Woodward, B., Duckworth, K., & Gutheil, J. (1993). The pharmacotherapist–psychotherapist collaboration. In J. M. Oldham, M. B. Riba, & A. Tasman (Eds.), *American Psychiatric Press review of psychiatry* (Vol. 12, pp. 731–649). Washington, DC: American Psychiatric Press.

Young, P. (1999). *Cognitive therapy for personality disorders: A schema-focused approach* (Rev. ed.). Sarasota, FL: Professional Resources Press.

Young, P., Klosko, J., & Weishaar, M. (2003). *Schema therapy: A practitioner's guide.* New York: Guilford Press.

Zautra, A., Burleson, M., Matt, K., Roth, S., & Burrows, L. (1994). Interpersonal stress, depression, and disease activity in rheumatoid arthritis. *Health Psychology, 13,* 139–148.

Zautra, A., & Manne, S. (1992). Coping with rheumatoid arthritis: A review of a decade of research. *Annals of Behavioral Medicine. 14,* 31–39.

Zimmerman, C., & Tansella, M. (1996). Psychological factors and physical illness in primary care: Promoting the biopsychosocial model in medical practice. *Journal of Psychosomatic Research, 40,* 352–358.

INDEX

health-focused counseling vs. health-focused psychotherapy for, 19
intolerance of, 34
issues unique to, 10–15
pain, suffering, and stigma in, 12–13
psychotherapeutic approaches to, 19–21
spiritual and religious issues in, 14
treatment of, 15–23
Clinical formulation, 107–108
  in case conceptualization, 131
  in diabetes case, 136
Cognitive–behavioral therapy (CBT), 20, 21–23
  empirical research on, 21–22
  for histrionic patient, 74
  for systemic lupus erythematosus, 63
  training materials for, 21
  for Type 1 diabetes, 22
Cognitive–behavioral treatment
  cognitive–behavioral therapy vs., 21
  by specialist vs. nonspecialist, 19
Cognitive methods, 161
Cognitive strategies
  for arthritis, 42
Cognitive therapy, 20
Collaborative relationship. *See also* Therapeutic relationship
  clinician's role in, 103
  countertransference in, 103–105
  engagement in, 102–103
  goals in, 110–111
Compliance
  borderline personality and, 90
  with diabetes treatment, 36
  with medication, enhancement of, 109
  noncompliance in systemic lupus erythematosus case, 154–155
  religious and spiritual beliefs and, 123
  trauma history effect on, 120
Comprehensive assessment process
  adequacy of health behaviors, 119
  in biopsychosocial therapy, 100
  explanatory model in, 105–106, 118
  exposure history in, 119
  family competence level and style, 122–123
  illness representation in, 117–118
  parental bond and adverse childhood experiences, 119–121
  patient resources in, 123–124
  pattern in, 106–107
  perpetuants in, 107

predisposition in, 107
presentation in, 106
religious and spiritual beliefs in, 123
self-capacities in, 124
treatment readiness in, 105
Compulsive personality
  behavioral and interpersonal styles of, 66
  developmental and etiological features of, 67
  emotional style of, 66
  experience of diabetes and, 69–70
  health-related dynamics in, 67–69
    demands of clinician, 67
    fear of loss of mastery, 68
    need for control in, 68–69
    preservation of defenses as key treatment goal, 69
  thinking style of, 66
Compulsive personality style, 194, 196
Constructivist perspective
  in biopsychosocial therapy, 100
Consultation session, 141
Conversion, 72
Coping
  components of, 29–30
  defined, 29
  in dependent personality, 77
Cost(s)
  of arthritis, 42
  of hypertension, 57
  personal, occupational, financial, 5
Counseling, 16
  health-focused, 19
  health promotion, 16, 17
  medical care, 15–16
  patient care, 15–16
Countertransference, 103
  in crisis phase, 104
  in integration phase, 105
  in resolution phase, 104–105
  in stabilization phase, 104
Crisis, 7
  assessment of, 126
  chronic fatigue syndrome example, 9
Cultural context
  of illness behavior, 33
  nonsupportive of persons with chronic illness, 34–35
Culture
  in perception and manifestation of health and illness, 33–34

in assessment process, 123–124

Pattern
in comprehensive assessment, 106–107

Pattern analysis
and case conceptualizations, 107–108
in diabetes case, 137, 138
as framework for case conceptualization, 134

Pattern change
and achievement of treatment outcomes, 108–109
as process goal, 111

Pattern maintenance and termination
as process goal, 111

Pattern recognition and analysis
as process goal, 111

Perpetuants
in comprehensive assessment, 107

Personality characteristics
appraisal of threat and, 30

Personality disorder
defined, 65, 122

Personality style
defined, 65, 122

Personal schemas
assessment of, 121

Physical activity
in cancer prevention, 47

Physician
case conceptualization of, 132–133
as fellow traveler vs. expert, 103

Pictorial Representation of Illness and Self Measure (PRISM), 129–130

Pilch, J., 11

Precipitants
in comprehensive assessment, 107

Predisposition
in comprehensive assessment, 107

Presentation
in comprehensive assessment, 106

Process goals, 110, 111

Pseudoseizures
epilepsy case, 161

Psychiatry
biopsychosocial model in, 26

Psychoeducational interventions, 109

Psychogenic seizures (pseudoseizures), 54
description of, 55–56
differentiation from epileptic seizures, 56
treatment of, 56–57

Psychological functioning, 27

Psychological stress
oxidative stress and, 32–33

Psychology
shift from psychological to biopsychosocial model in, 16

Psychosocial interventions, 101

Psychosocial model
interface with biological variables, 30
stress and coping in, 29–30

Psychosocial treatments
for systemic lupus erythematosus, 63

Psychotherapeutic interventions, 101

Psychotherapy
health-focused, 16, 19
for irritable bowel syndrome, 20–21, 60
meta-analyses of, 22–23
for psychogenic seizures (pseudoseizures), 56–57

Racial minorities
prevalence of chronic illness in, 5

Readiness for treatment
assessment of, 124–125

Reframing
in epilepsy case, 184, 185

Relapse
cyclicity of, 110
prevention of, 109

Relationship. *See also* Collaborative relationship; Therapeutic relationship
primacy of, in biopsychosocial therapy, 100

Relaxation training
for histrionic patient, 74

Religious beliefs
in assessment process, 123

Resolution, 8
assessment of, 126
chronic fatigue syndrome example, 9–10

Rheumatoid arthritis
models of, 28

Sarcoma
defined, 45

Schemas
defined, 121
maladaptive, 121, 161

Schema therapy, 121

Search for meaning, 14, 15

Secondary gain
in borderline personality, 91

ABOUT THE AUTHOR

Len Sperry, MD, PhD, has practiced psychotherapy with people who have health-related issues for more than 20 years. He is currently professor and a doctoral program coordinator at Florida Atlantic University as well as clinical professor of psychiatry and behavioral medicine at the Medical College of Wisconsin. A fellow of the American Psychological Association, he is also a distinguished fellow of the American Psychiatric Association and a fellow of the American College of Preventive Medicine. In addition to being a diplomate in clinical psychology of the American Board of Professional Psychology, he is a diplomate of the American Board of Psychiatry and Neurology and the American Board of Preventive Medicine. He is listed in *Who's Who in America, Best Doctors in America,* and *Guide to America's Top Physicians* and is a recipient of two lifetime achievement awards, including the Harry Levinson Award from the American Psychological Association. Among his 300 publications are 50 professional books including the recently published *Handbook of Diagnosis and Treatment of DSM–IV–TR Personality Disorders, Second Edition,* and *Health Promotion and Health Counseling: Effective Counseling and Psychotherapeutic Strategies, Second Edition.*